ALZHEIMER'S
STORIES

ALZHEIMER'S STORIES

ALZHEIMER'S STORIES

A CAREGIVER'S GUIDE TO MISMATCHED OUTFITS, GOOFY HAIR AND BEER FOR BREAKFAST.

KAREN FAVO WALSH

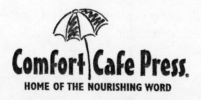

Comfort Cafe Press.
HOME OF THE NOURISHING WORD

ISBN 1-59113-418-8

Join our Alzheimer's newsletter group:
Alzheimers_Stories-subscribe@yahoogroups.com.

Copies of this publication available in print or electronic format:
www.booklocker.com.

This book is for those who choose the journey. Special thanks to my tour guide Billie, and my travel companions: Frank, Charlie, Emily and Daniel.

ALZHEIMER'S STORIES

THE STORIES

INTRODUCTION – 1

ONE: A Slow Descent – 3

TWO: Seizures – 10

THREE: Watch Your Step – 18

FOUR: Creative Cuisine for Cats and People – 22

FIVE: Advice for Houseguests – 25

SIX: What About Hygiene? – 29

SEVEN: Our Daily Grief – 36

EIGHT: Adult Day Care – 39

NINE: First Day in Day Care – 46

TEN: Trouble on Day Three – 50

ELEVEN: The Struggle to Shampoo – 54

TWELVE: Support Group – 59

THIRTEEN: Kicked Out of Day Care – 66

FOURTEEN: The Next Transition: Assisted Living – 74

FIFTEEN: Billie's New Home – 83

SIXTEEN: The Snapshot Visit – 91

SEVENTEEN: Emotional Whiplash – 96

EIGHTEEN: The Odyssey – 108

NINETEEN: A Bedtime Story – 119

TWENTY: Heart Strings – 122

EPILOGUE – 125

APPENDIX A:
   The Ten Warning Signs of Alzheimer's Disease with
   Examples of Billie's Specific Behaviors – 129

ACKNOWLEDGMENTS – 137

Do you suspect someone you love suffers from Alzheimer's Disease (AD)? Curious behaviors surface long before an official diagnosis. Is your person hiding your shoes, repeating stories, wandering?

You're not alone. The worldwide estimate by Alzheimer's Disease International is eighteen million people currently have AD. Millions more are caregivers.

Alzheimer's Stories is full of honest, intimate details about Alzheimer's. Its short, relevant chapters provide fast advice to time-starved caregivers. I hope this book helps you find the magic moments hidden inside this incredible disease. —K.F.W.

ALZHEIMER'S STORIES

CHAPTER ONE

A Slow Descent

"She's at the top of the hill, about to fall down it."
— Neurologist's description of Billie, July 27, 1999

*B*illie sits back on her heels and squints at the setting Florida sun. Her hand paints a brown line of dirt across her forehead as she wipes perspiration above her gray eyebrows. "I don't always understand conversations or directions," she says.

I kneel on the ground next to her. My toddler, Emily, plops down beside me.

"What do you mean?" I ask.

"What I hear isn't always what people say." She yanks the weeds around an unruly red hibiscus. "Oh, don't listen to me. I'm crazy." She forces a laugh.

ALZHEIMER'S STORIES

"No, you're not." I pull weeds, too. "Your hearing aid should help. Don't worry."

Billie stands and brushes dirt off her kneecaps. She shakes her head.

Billie is a retired librarian and one-time preacher's wife. She and my father-in-law, Frank, have been companions since 1976. Practicing Buddhists, they are former hippies who marched for civil rights, Native Americans, feminism and the environment. Now, they attend museums, lectures, concerts and new restaurants. They spend winter here in Florida, and summer on Saginaw Bay in Michigan.

Emily and Billie wander away from me. Hand-in-hand they stroll across the yard gathering fallen twigs and palm fronds. Sunlight bounces across Emily's yellow curls and brightens Billie's tentative smile.

Eighteen months earlier, in May 1986, Billie sat by my bed on the high-risk maternity floor of Bayfront Medical Center in St. Petersburg. Twenty-six years-old and eight-and-a-half months pregnant, I was in the hospital for complete bed rest. Pregnancy-induced hypertension.

My family was far away in Pennsylvania. My husband Charlie had to work all day. Billie's frequent visits cheered me during an uncomfortable attachment to a fetal monitor, catheter and IV. She delivered books, magazines and a deluxe green and white striped diaper bag. She rubbed my back, told funny stories and assured me our baby would be healthy.

Billie was with me when I left recovery and held Emily for the first time, three days after her birth. A week later,

Charlie, Emily and I went home as a new family. Billie cooked meals, babysat so I could nap, and embraced Emily as her own granddaughter.

Now, Billie needs comfort from me. Her expensive new ear piece can't solve her auditory problem. Something in her fifty-nine-year-old brain scrambles information, with or without the aid in her ear.

Four weeks later, Billie loses her high-tech hearing aid. As time passes, the problem becomes more and more serious. Within four years, she misplaces larger objects.

"Billie's at the mall and can't find the car. Can you drive me there?" My father-in-law, Frank, chuckles over the phone.

"Sure, we'll come get you," I say. "I just painted clown faces on the kids, so we look silly."

My five-year-old, Emily, a blonde clown in a tie-dyed sundress and pink plastic sandals leads us into Tyrone Square Mall. Daniel, my three-year-old blue-eyed boy, follows her. They swing their arms and smile at the Saturday shoppers. I walk behind them, next to Frank. The paint spatter in my auburn hair and on my black shorts identifies me as the clowns' escort. Frank's glasses, gray hair and beard don't resemble a clown, but his green socks and yellow suspenders add color.

Our search party hustles through the mall. Daniel stops to press his red clown nose against a glass booth in the concourse.

"I want a pretzel," he says to a teenage boy tying dough in a knot.

"Come on, Daniel." I take his hand. "We have to find

Grandma Billie. We'll eat later." As we pass Burdines, my eyes lock on the summer business suits in the same way Daniel eyed the pretzels.

At the JCPenney-Dairy Queen intersection, I stretch my neck to view the pay phones in front of the Ritz Camera store. Billie is there, dressed in an Everglades tee shirt and faded jean shorts. A silver pony tail hangs down the center of her back. Only her eyes move as she scans the weekend shoppers for a familiar face. Her Birkenstock sandals stick to the floor in the precise location she described to Frank. "I'll stand by the phone until you get here."

Billie's shoulders straighten when she sees us. A grin replaces her tight-lipped frown. "Well, look who's here! Look at your faces!" She hugs the clowns as if they were away at the circus. Her green eyes fill with tears. "Oh, Frank."

"Don't worry. We'll find the car," he says. "We always park by Dillard's. We'll look there first." He pats her shoulder. Emily and Daniel each grab one of her hands.

Ten minutes later, Billie and Frank reunite with their car outside the main entrance to Dillard's. They follow us home. I paint clown faces on them, too. The face paint can't hide the growing seriousness of Billie's memory loss.

Billie develops coping skills to deal with her impairment. "You're right about that" or "I'll say" serve her in any conversation. Her forgetfulness leads to repetition. During Sunday dinners at our house, Billie repeats herself six times during one meal. We always pretend the story is new.

Her next symptom is wandering. It grows from nuisance to major problem in a year. Billie disappears at the grocery store, the movies and restaurants. Friends and relatives begin to chaperone her on all excursions. We don't lose Billie as often, but we do still lose her.

On a balmy March afternoon, music, food and people mingle in the city's waterfront park. Frank and Billie watch Irish dancers at the 1998 St. Petersburg International Folk Festival. Grills sizzle and grease fryers bubble as gyros, funnel cakes and egg rolls cook under fifty white tents. Sweet and savory smells tickle our noses. A relaxed afternoon turns tense with one question: "Where's Billie?"

Family and friends huddle in a tight circle.

"Where can she be?"

"She's probably watching the bagpipes."

"Do you think she left the park?"

"I hope she isn't scared."

"How will we ever find her? There must be ten thousand people here."

By foot, bike and car we search around performers, families, teenage couples and retirees. Three times we separate, explore and reassemble. It's a futile hour-long search. When we don't know what else to do, we call Frank's house.

"I wondered where everyone was," Billie says into the phone. "What are you doing?"

We can only guess how she traveled three miles from the festival to home.

In July 1999, Charlie, the kids and I visit Billie and Frank at the Michigan house Frank's family built on Saginaw Bay in 1911. When we arrive, they resemble over-weight, sleep-

7

deprived zombies. Nocturnal bouts of paranoia and disorientation cause Billie to wake Frank several times every night.

"Billie gets up three or four times a night," Frank says, "Sometimes she's frightened, sometimes she's hungry." He shrugs. "We probably eat lunch two or three times a day now. I don't argue when she forgets her last meal was an hour earlier. It's just easier to eat again."

Two of Billie's three grown children live in Michigan. Jenni and her family live twenty minutes down the road in Bay City. Craig's home is in Ann Arbor, two hours away.

During our visit, Frank, Billie, her kids and I drive into Bay City for Billie's appointment with a neurologist. Dr. Bong Jung examines her and announces she has Alzheimer's Disease. He tells us, "She's at the top of the hill, about to fall down it."

The next morning, Frank and I join Craig and Jenni in a meeting with a Bay County healthcare worker. We schedule twice weekly visits with a nurse's aide to help Billie shower. The home health visits end after two attempts. Billie refuses to cooperate.

Throughout Billie's cognitive decline, Frank is patient and accepting. "Billie doesn't remember yesterday, and she doesn't worry about tomorrow. So, what's the problem?" he asks.

The problem is Alzheimer's causes absurd and potentially dangerous situations. When Frank has a serious asthma attack, Billie calls 4-1-1 instead of 9-1-1. What will happen when she forgets 4-1-1?

For twenty-three years, Billie and Frank have spent their

summers in Michigan and winters in Florida. After Billie's Alzheimer's diagnosis, Charlie and I prepare Frank's home in St. Petersburg for year-round living. We want Frank and Billie near us.

In November 1999, I resign from work. It's a dramatic switch from the fast lane of business to the surreal, meandering path of Alzheimer's.

It is time to help Billie negotiate her way down the hill.

CHAPTER TWO

Seizures

"This is ridiculous."
— Billie

On day fourteen of my caregiving career, Frank calls at seven in the morning. "Karen, can you come now? Billie is having a seizure."

In six minutes, I'm across town in the upstairs bedroom of his 1930s Craftsman-style home.

"Oh, here it comes again," Billie cries. I sit on the bed next to her. Antique springs creak as she leans over the side of the carved walnut bed and vomits into a wastebasket.

Billie wraps her arms around her stomach and winces. Her cycle of pain, perspiration, vomit and expelled mucus ends in a deep sleep.

I push sweaty gray hair away from her closed eyes. "What happened?" I ask.

Frank shifts his weight from left foot to right. He strokes his beard, then fidgets with his eyeglasses.

"I may have given Billie an extra dose of medicine." He stares at me with worried brown eyes. "It's possible I gave her two pills last night."

Donepezil hydrochloride is a drug prescribed to relieve anxiety and paranoia caused by Alzheimer's. Billie's dosage is one pill before bed.

Downstairs a wooden screen door slams. A familiar voice calls, "Hello? Anyone here?" Frank descends to tell Betsy, a family friend, what's happening. I hear them chant their morning Buddhist prayers a few minutes later.

In the next hour, Billie suffers three painful cycles. Her face is as white as the washcloth I use to wipe her steamy forehead. Perspiration saturates her pink flannel nightgown. The wet bed sheet clings like a magnet to the plastic mattress cover.

"Lie on your side Billie. I'll rub your back."

"Ohh-kay," she moans.

Soon, she falls asleep. As I rise to rinse the washcloth in the adjacent bathroom, Billie's body jerks. Her right arm jumps from her side and hits the bed stand. A glass of water crashes to the hardwood floor. Billie's head snaps back. Her body stiffens. Her green eyes roll until her sockets are white.

"Oh God! Billie!"

I shake her shoulders.

"BILLIE!"

No response.

"Call 9-1-1," I scream. "Call 9-1-1."

Frank and Betsy appear. Betsy is on the cordless phone with a 9-1-1 dispatcher. Questions and answers fly across the room. Betsy disconnects. "They're coming."

I shake Billie. "Billie, wake up Billie."

Faint sirens.

Loud sirens.

Betsy races down the stairs to meet the paramedics. Billie stirs. She groans and opens her eyes.

Two paramedics and a fireman stomp up the stairs. Metal cases filled with medical paraphernalia crash to the floor. The room is crowded. The sloped ceiling feels claustrophobic. Billie looks like a worn-out rag doll tossed on the bed.

A thirty-ish EMS worker shines a penlight at Billie's tiny pupils. "Hi. I'm Liz, a paramedic. Can you tell me what you're feeling?"

"I don't know." Billie looks at each stranger's face.

"She has Alzheimer's," I say.

Liz adjusts her blond ponytail. She grabs Billie's chin with her thumb and two fingers, then leans forward. "Do you hurt?" she shouts.

"I don't know." Billie wiggles her chin free.

I say, "She clutches her stomach and groans, then she vomits. And, she's burning up."

Liz talks into a radio attached to her shoulder. "We'll take her to emergency so they can examine her."

Liz and her partner Dave lift Billie's plump, pear-shaped body into a transport chair. Before the seat belt is buckled,

Billie seizes again. Dark-haired, muscular Dave catches Billie before she falls. He lays her stiff body on the bed. Liz monitors vital signs.

In ten seconds, Billie regains consciousness. Dave and Liz secure her in the transport chair and carry her downstairs to the ambulance. They drive six blocks to St. Anthony's Hospital.

Four and a half hours later, in a chilly emergency room cubicle, Billie sits on the edge of the bed dressed in a hospital gown and gray slipper socks. Her hair, recently cut short for easy care, sticks out in all directions. She is one of six patients in the ER.

The beds form a semi-circle around the nurses' desk. Each cubicle contains a wall of medical instruments. Blue nylon drapes swing around the beds like a shower curtain for visual privacy. There is no sound barrier.

Other patients, in assorted stages of emergency, each have a friend or family member with them. Everyone whispers a collective "there, there, everything will be okay."

Our nurse whips the blue curtain aside. In a sharp voice she reports, "Nothing is wrong with Billie. She seems fine now. She can go home. Doctor signed off on it."

"Really?" I look from the nurse to Billie. "Well. Okay Billie, let's get your clothes on."

The nurse vanishes without closing the curtain.

Billie leans against the bed as I pull on her pants. Before her foot is in the second leg, she seizes for the fourth time today. Her five-foot-three-inch frame stiffens. She falls sideways.

"Nurse!" I catch Billie's falling body. "NURSE!"
The nurse appears, and together we lay Billie lengthwise on the bed.

Fifteen seconds later, her eyelids flutter open.

"She's not going anywhere," the nurse barks. "I'll call the neurologist to come look at her." She pulls the sheet to Billie's waist then rushes away.

I sit on the bed next to Billie. We hold hands and wait.

"Frank's waiting for us to come outside," I say.

"Why are we here?" Billie asks.

"You fainted and the doctors want to make sure you're okay." We repeat the conversation seven times before the neurologist arrives.

"Hi, I'm Doctor Lin." She glances at her clipboard. "Are you Billie?"

"Yes." Billie smiles.

Dr. Lin taps her pen on the clipboard. "I'm going to ask you a few questions, Billie. I want you to remember this green pen for me, okay?"

"Sure." Billie swishes her legs back and forth under the sheet.

"Do you know where you are?"

"Right here."

"Do you know who is with you?"

Billie grimaces.

"Who is the president?"

"Oh, that guy," she laughs.

"Do you remember what color my pen is?" Dr. Lin taps Billie's arm with the green ballpoint.

"Sure. What now?"

Dr. Lin orders an MRI, carotid artery ultrasound and a CAT scan. Then she tells us, "Today is Saturday. These tests aren't performed on the weekend, so Billie will be admitted and have the tests on Monday."

Hours later, in a pink room with a floral wallpaper border, the mood grows tense. The cozy mauve visitor chairs don't fool Billie. The industrial linoleum floor, hospital bed and blue privacy curtain trigger her internal alarms.

"This isn't home," Billie says, "Why am I here?"

"Because you fainted." I stroke her arm. "The doctors want to make sure you're okay."

"Why can't I go home? I have a nice home. This is ridiculous!"

"You fainted and the doctors want to run tests."

Billie throws back her bed covers. "I have to go to the bathroom."

"There's a catheter hooked to you." I tuck the blanket under her hips. "You don't need to get up."

"Why are we here?" Billie pounds her fists on the bed.

"We're waiting for the doctor."

She kicks her feet under the sheet. "Why can't I go home? THIS IS RIDICULOUS!"

A skittish, pregnant nurse darts into the room. She lisps, "Bil-wie, can I take your tem-pa-ture? We need to do this. Open your mouth."

Billie bops her in the nose. A few minutes later, Billie punches another nurse in the arm as she delivers a dinner tray. Two strikes and Billie is in arm restraints.

She scrunches her face. "#%*@ this!" She struggles to free her arms. "Can't you get me out of this?" she asks.

"I don't know how," I say.

"That's stupid." Her mouth twists with rage. "You're stupid. Stupid!" She curses again and again, and again.

"Don't get upset Billie," I say.

"Why not?" she hisses, "You're upset!"

Ten silent minutes later, Billie forgets. She makes funny faces at the nurses' backs. We discuss things and people we like.

Patrice, the pregnant nurse, returns at eight with Billie's bedtime sedative. "Oh-Oh-kay Bil-wie," she stammers. "Here's sum-thing for you to eat." She positions a tiny white pill on Billie's tongue.

Billie spits the pill onto the bed.

"Oh. No, no, no, Bil-wie. You need to SWALLOW it." Patrice pretends to put the pill in her mouth and swallow. "Like this," she says, "Mmmm."

"Come on, Billie," I say, "You'll feel better."

Billie sticks out her tongue at me. Patrice drops the pill onto it. Billie chomps it. She chews until it's gone. Soon, she is her sweet, gentle self.

"This is a nice place," she says. "Is it your house? Did Charlie fix it up?"

"Yes he did, do you like it?" I ask.

"He did a beautiful job." Billie looks at the floor to my right and smiles. "How sweet. Whose dogs are those?"

"Those are our dogs." I smile at the imaginary animals.

"Pretty." Billie's eyelids flutter, droop and close.

More sedatives make Billie's three tests possible on Monday. She remains groggy that night, but the nurses don't remove her restraints. On Tuesday morning, the doctor delivers the test results. "Billie is healthy except for the Alzheimer's. There is no reason for her seizures. We don't know what caused them." Billie is right. This is ridiculous.

CHAPTER THREE

Watch Your Step

"It's easy to see things once you know where you are."
— Billie

Outside, Billie scurries past the kitchen window, across the side yard and into the alley.

I wonder aloud, "How does a seventy-two-year-old woman bent in half, walk so fast?" My knife clatters into the ceramic sink as I drop lunch preparations to chase her.

Alzheimer's fogs Billie's mind. Sedatives she received during her recent three-day hospital stay make her body bend at a right angle. It's not a good combination.

According to Billie's doctor, sedatives often have a "second life" or residual effect. In older people the symptoms can last days after dosing ends.

"Normal posture will return," the doctor assures me, "when the meds are completely out of her system."

Until Billie is five-foot-three again, I must make sure she doesn't topple forward.

When I reach the alley, Billie is four blocks ahead, turning right onto Fifteenth Avenue. I race down the alley and find her just past the corner. She stands in the street facing the curb. Her nose is inches above the ground. She scratches her neck and stares at the granite street edging.

"Hey Billie, whatcha doing?" I ask.

She points to the steep incline of lush manicured lawn above the curb. "I want to get there," she says.

"Let's go over here." I wave at the adjacent driveway with an easier grade.

"No, no. I can do it. But..."

"Then let me help you." I put an arm around her shoulders.

Billie aims her index finger at a giant pile of dog dirt in the grass in front of us. "Watch your step," she warns.

I smell it before I see it. "Okay. Let's try the driveway instead."

"Oh no, no." Billie shakes her head. She draws a deep breath. "One, two, three, let's go."

Pushing me for momentum, she puts her right foot on the curb. Her second step reaches the grass. When her right leg swings forward again, Billie doesn't notice her foot lands on the mound. She bends closer to the ground and speeds her gait.

"Whoa, don't go so fast." I grab her arm. "You'll fall if you don't slow down."

"Okay," she sighs. She strolls for thirty seconds, then races again.

At the corner, I suggest the shortest route home.

"No." Billie freezes in place. "We have to go this way."

I look at her determined face. An argument makes as little sense as taking the long way home. When she yanks my arm, I cooperate. We retrace our steps until we're back in the alley.

Sweat dances across Billie's forehead. On this seventy-five degree day she wears two tee shirts, a green cotton pullover, and my father-in-law's gray wool cardigan which hangs to her knees. All this is over a pair of black pants. Layered clothing is another symptom of Alzheimer's. Billie's brain can no longer determine appropriate dress. She forgets she has a shirt on and adds a second and often a third one.

I coax her out of the wool cardigan when we pause to rest. We walk four more feet before she wants to remove her oversized pullover. "Too hot."

Billie wipes her brow with the sleeve, then disappears inside her sweater. A muffled "uh-oh" reaches my ears. I plant my feet in the gravel. It's a struggle to keep Billie upright. Her head pushes into one sleeve, pauses, then enters the other sleeve. She's stuck.

"Oh God," I mutter. Our feet kick loose stones around the alley. Twice, we shuffle in a full circle. My left arm hugs Billie's waist as I pull the sweater loose with my right hand. A warm waft of her perspiration fills my nose as she appears outside her sweater.

"There you are," I say.

Billie squints at the sun. "Here," she tosses the pullover at my face, "that's better."

"Thanks a lot." I pull her arm like a lever to straighten her. A quick glance up and down the alley reveals no witnesses to our antics. We resume our journey.

Slow. Race. Repeat.

Slow. Race. Repeat.

A block from home I ask, "Billie, why are you walking so fast?"

She stops to look up at me from her hunched position. "I'm so tired," she pants, "I want to get home quick so I can take a nap."

CHAPTER FOUR

Creative Cuisine
for Cats and People

"People food can hurt animals."
— Billie

As I crack and remove shells from hard-boiled eggs, Billie collects them to feed to her cats.

"I don't think cats like egg shells," I say.

"That's the problem with your generation," Billie sneers. She opens the kitchen screen door and puts the bowl of shells on the back porch. "Here kitties. Here kitty, kitty."

Two gray striped cats rush the blue dish. Billie smiles as they sniff the egg shells. The cats stare at Billie, then slink away.

Billie puts both hands on her hips. "I'm the only one who

knows how to feed cats." She returns to the kitchen and gathers buttered toast and orange slices. She adds them to the back porch buffet. Again, the cats scurry to the food. They sniff, meow, leave.

An hour later, Billie places an unopened can of cat food on the back steps. She sets a half-eaten banana floating in a bowl of coffee next to it.

Billie is dangerous in the kitchen as her disease progresses. There are safety concerns, such as leaving the stove on, but a more common hazard is she'll serve a peanut butter and dish soap sandwich. Billie washes dishes with pumice soap and places them in the drying rack without a rinse. She uses dish towels as Kleenex for her constantly dripping nose.

I hide the towels. I wash every dish and utensil before use. All inedible cleansers are hidden in the detached garage studio. The effort to retrieve them is worth peace of mind. No one wants food seasoned with window cleaner, furniture polish or laundry detergent.

Today, lunch is tuna salad sandwiches. I drain two cans of tuna and put the contents into a mixing bowl.

"Billie, do you want to mix in the mayonnaise?"

"Sure." She stands next to me at the kitchen counter.

I hand her a large spoon. She heaps six generous spoonfuls of mayonnaise on the tuna. She whistles as she stirs. I cut carrots into finger food. Billie grabs the carrots and drops them one at a time into her tuna soup.

My husband Charlie arrives. "What's for lunch?" He peers over Billie's shoulder to see the bowl in front of her. "Yuck, what's that?"

Billie grins. "Hi, Charlie." She tosses in more carrots. Charlie's eyes question me.

"I can make it edible," I say, "Don't worry."

"No way." He opens the kitchen door. "I'll grab fast food on my way back to work."

Billie sets spoons around the table. I doctor her creation with herbs, spices and two additional cans of tuna. I extract the carrots and replace them with chopped celery. While Billie calls Frank to lunch, I sneak a can of cat food outside to the felines.

Billie, Frank and I munch our tuna sandwiches and rinsed carrot sticks. After two bites of her sandwich, Billie leaves her seat. She pulls honey, ketchup and a jar of green olives from the refrigerator. She arranges everything on the table, "for whoever wants these."

At the end of the meal, Billie cradles a loaf of bread. "How about this for dessert?"

I clear dishes into the sink. "I brought our favorite poppy seed cake for dessert today."

The screen door slams as I reach for the cake hidden on top of the refrigerator. "It's gone." I look at Frank, alone at the table.

He points his index finger at the backyard. Billie sits in a lawn chair. She hand-feeds our favorite poppy seed cake to her two cats, plus a calico stray from the neighborhood.

Like the cats, Frank and I never know what Billie will serve us. But because it pleases her, we accept her creative cuisine even when we don't dare eat it.

CHAPTER FIVE

Advice for Houseguests

"Things disappear fast around here."
— Karen

I give this advice to everyone who visits Billie and Frank: "Never put anything down if you want to see it again. It only takes a second for something to disappear." Most guests don't believe me until after they are victims of Billie's Alzheimer's Disease.

When I arrive for my daily visit, Frank and his friend, Dick are in the detached studio. Inside the converted garage are a lithographic press, two drafting tables, a built-in countertop and heaps of colorful art supplies. Mounds of rubber stamps, ink pads and gadgets cover all available space. The smell of old books hangs in the air.

Frank sits on a tall stool at his drafting table. "Well look, it's the redhead. Hello, Karen." He swishes a calligraphy pen across paper.

Dick, Frank's longtime friend and lawyer, is in town to prepare tax returns. He sits at the counter surrounded by stacks of books. His golf shirt and pressed pants look lawyerly, but his gray hair points north in three directions. He squints at an official document six inches from his tan face.

"Where are your glasses?" I ask.

Dick clears his throat. "In the house. I'll get them later."

"Oh." I raise an eyebrow. "I'll go say hello to Mary and Billie and let you two work."

Inside the house, Dick's wife Mary darts around the living room. She tosses couch pillows, magazines and newspapers. Billie mimics each action.

"What's going on?" I ask as Mary speeds towards the fireplace.

"Dick put his glasses on the coffee table this morning. Five minutes later, they were gone." Her blue eyes survey the room. "I've searched for an hour and can't find them."

She waves her arms. "Dick can't see without his glasses."

"Okay." I glance around the room. "Billie hides things in bags and drawers, and behind stuff on the shelves. We have to look everywhere."

Mary studies the ceiling-to-floor bookshelves in the dining room. "Okay, then." She runs her fingers through her hair and faces the rows of books.

Billie asks, "How about this?" She plops a floppy white

canvas hat on her head, tugs at both sides and grins. Circling Mary, she offers a blue coffee mug and *The New Yorker* magazine. "Do you want this?" Billie picks up a pink dish towel. "Is this it?"

Mary looks at each object and shakes her head. "No. Thanks Billie, no."

Billie wanders through the kitchen and out the back door. Her barefoot figure waddles down three porch steps towards the garage studio. Still holding the towel, she plucks fruit from a citrus tree in the backyard. She tucks the orange and towel among Frank's art supplies as she enters the studio.

I hunt in the kitchen for Dick's glasses. Behind the microwave, I find two saltine crackers in a used napkin. Old mail stuffed into a year-old birthday card hides under books on the table. A toothbrush, four clothespins and a handkerchief fill a dirty white sock. The sock is in a raisin bran cereal box on the pantry shelf.

As Mary searches the first floor, I climb the stairs to the bedroom Billie and Frank share. In a yellow overnight bag Billie constantly packs and unpacks are more clothespins, an empty tube of toothpaste, Kleenex, a bar of soap and the book *I'll Never Get Lost Again*. There are no eyeglasses.

A small brightly colored drawstring purse, hanging from the towel rack in the attached bathroom, catches my eye. *Ah ha!* I think, *This has to be it. It's the perfect size for eyeglasses.*

I grab the woven purse and reach inside. Instead of glasses, my fingers find an egg salad sandwich. An egg salad sandwich? Yesterday's lunch leftovers. Thank goodness it's in a plastic baggie.

After a thorough search of the second floor, I return downstairs. Mary looks hopeful, then puzzled, as I descend holding the sandwich.

Forty-five minutes later, we find Dick's glasses wedged between books on the piano in the living room.

Our game of hide-and-seek isn't over. By two-thirty, Frank and I search for Billie's left shoe, a bottle of marinade and a new grapefruit knife. We find the shoe.

Frank writes "marinade" and "knife" on our posted list of missing items. Today the tally includes a razor cord, the sun shade for the car, Frank's Tampa Bay Devil Rays windbreaker and the television remote control.

Maybe, we'll find them tomorrow.

CHAPTER SIX

What About Hygiene?

"You're so stupid. I can't even explain it to you."
— Billie

*B*illie putters in the yard every day. She clears fallen branches under the sixty-year-old oaks. She rearranges heavy Adirondack-style lawn furniture. Dressed in multiple layers of clothing, she sweats in the midday sun. Her bare feet collect black dirt.

BATHING

The many steps to taking a bath can overwhelm an Alzheimer's patient. Medical resources suggest soothing music and slow explanations to ease the patient into a bathtub. The idea is to break the process into small steps so it's easier for the patient to understand.

Since Frank won't bathe her, and Billie won't bathe herself, I'm her best hope for good hygiene.

This morning, Billie and I have three hours to ourselves. Frank will be in the garage studio with his calligraphy group from nine until noon.

Billie follows me into the downstairs bathroom. It's a spacious room with a ten foot ceiling. Tiny rectangular floor tiles match larger peach ceramic squares that climb four feet up the walls.

On the far wall, the bathtub is framed by an arch. A large frosted window provides light and privacy. On the right is the original sink with two faucets. Beside the sink is a new, tall "senior friendly" toilet, advertised as easy seating for the elderly.

"You know, Billie," I pull my hair into a pony tail, "I think it's time for you to take a bath, to clean up."
I push my shirt sleeves past my elbows.

"Oh no," Billie answers, "You go ahead."

"I showered this morning. It's your turn."

"Okay." She strolls out of the bathroom.

Often if I wait a few minutes and try again, Billie's resistance disappears. I push the flamingo print shower curtain aside and turn the faucet in the bathtub.

Billie reappears. "You don't need to do that."

"I want to help you take a bath."

"What are you doing?" she asks.

"Running a bath for you. Look at your feet. They're dirty, why don't we wash them?"

"That's dumb." She leaves.

Although I'm two inches taller, Billie outweighs me by forty-five pounds. She looks harmless, but I know her superhuman strength to resist. I can't force her to take a bath. I clean the bathroom, add hot water to the tub and wait for her to return.

"Well, look who's here!" Billie rediscovers me.

"Hey Billie, ready for your bath?"

I reach for her sweater and coax it off. My babbling narrative distracts her. I remove the first of her two tee shirts. Ripe body odor assaults my nose. "Let's get this last shirt off so you can take a nice, warm bath."

"No, no, no." Billie applies a death grip to my arms.

Like studio wrestlers in a stalemate, we shift from one foot to the other. I swing side-to-side, but can't shake her grasp.

"Don't you want that dirt off your feet?" I ask.

Billie grits her teeth. She dares me with her eyes.

I laugh. "Why am I trying to reason with you?"

She hugs her shirt. "No."

"Okay, okay." I rub the red finger impressions on my arms. "Never mind."

An hour later, with past attempts forgotten, we're back in the bathroom.

"Come with me, Billie. I put a folded towel on the closed toilet. Holding both of her hands, I ease her onto the seat. "Sit here."

"I'm going to use this warm washcloth to clean you, okay?" I press the cloth on her forearm. "See, isn't that nice?"

Billie doesn't resist. I bend her elbows one at a time and ease her arms out of her sleeves. The dirty tee shirt hangs like a necklace around her neck.

"Hold this towel around your shoulders." I pull the shirt over her head. "It'll keep you warm."

"No." Billie protests. She grabs for the shirt as I toss it across the room.

I wash each hand, wrist and arm, then lift the towel to bathe her shoulders. Dirt hides inside the wrinkles of her neck. The wash cloth stays warm with repeated rinses in the sink of hot soapy water.

As I wash her chest and back, Billie shivers.

"You don't need to do that," she says.

I hug her with the towel and dry with a vigorous back rub. Together we chant, "Aaaahhhh oooohhhh eeewww."

She laughs.

"Let's put this shirt on." I slip a fresh top over her head and pull it to her waist.

She looks at me with sad eyes.

"Now, about these feet. We'd better work on them next, don't you think?"

"I don't think so." Billie tucks her feet around the base of the toilet.

"Let's try," I say. I refill the sink with fresh soapy water.

Billie stands.

"Sit down, Billie," I guide her back to her seat. "We're almost done. Just one more minute."

I kneel in front of her filthy feet. "Mmmm. Doesn't this vanilla soap smell good?" I hold the washcloth under her nose.

"Ah-huh." Billie giggles as I slide the cloth between her toes. Her foot jerks. I fall backwards on my butt. She laughs out loud.

"You think that's funny?" I stand.

"Yep." She rises from her seat.

Billie grabs the waistband of her pants as I unzip them. "Oh, no." Her weathered face crumbles.

"It's okay, Billie. I need to wash the rest of you."

"No. No," she cries.

I hug Billie and pat her back. As she returns my hug, I push the pants off her hips.

"Hold these panties." I hand clean underwear to her. "We'll change you. Then, I'll help you get dressed."

Billie is agitated, then agreeable, then agitated again as I remove yesterday's underwear and wash her. Soon, she smells like vanilla instead of old sweat.

I attempt immersion bathing again the next week. It doesn't work. I decide to redefine bathing as sponge baths, washing Billie after she uses the bathroom, and a daily change of clothes.

DENTAL

Billie applies toothpaste directly from the tube onto her front teeth. Her face is inches from the bathroom mirror. She pushes the tube back and forth across her pearly whites.

"Come look at Billie," I whisper to Frank, "You'll want to know your toothpaste's condition."

Frank peeks around the doorway at Billie. He moans, "I guess I'll use baking soda for toothpaste from now on."

At the dental office, Billie's hygienist laments, "It's so sad, she used to take such good care of her teeth." She turns to me. "You must brush Billie's teeth twice a day."

"I'll do my best," I promise.

Billie behaves in the dentist's office. At home when I brush her teeth, it's different.

I load her toothbrush with paste, add a splash of water and aim for her toothy grin. She smiles at me and then at herself in the mirror over the bathroom sink.

"Grrr." Billie clenches her teeth.

"Open up. I'll help you brush," I say.

"Okay."

As she answers, I tuck the toothbrush under her lips and move it towards her molars.

"Ooww. Ouch. Billie, stop!"

Billie's eyes widen at my cry. Her teeth grip my finger, thumb and the toothbrush.

"Open your mouth," I beg. "Quick. Say something."

"Stop bothering me."

INCONTINENCE

A minor problem for years, Billie's incontinence escalates into a major problem.

Some mornings, I find panties drying on the kitchen paper towel rack or porch railing. My nose leads me to dirty underwear hidden in bookcases, wastebaskets and under her bed.

When Billie's incontinence is no longer intermittent, I buy disposable adult diapers. I remove her cotton panties and replace them with the adult diapers.

"These ugly things aren't underwear," she grumbles to Frank before I arrive the next morning. She refuses to wear them. After less than a day, I realize Billie's choice of no underwear is far worse than dirty underwear.

***

I haven't found a secret to easy hygiene. Some days are okay, other days are incredibly gross. For now, frequent hand-washing, sponge baths, regular trips to the hair salon and dentist, plus daily laundry are my best solution.

CHAPTER SEVEN

Our Daily Grief

"Frank is dead."
— Billie

Tears follow wrinkle detours as they slide down Billie's cheeks. Reddish-brown circles surround her tired eyes. Tiny pupils lack focus. She is lost in a world where emotions are real, even when the facts aren't.

"Betty is dead," she sobs.

I wrap my arm around her shoulders and squeeze. Her sister isn't dead.

Alzheimer's causes Billie daily grief. Health professionals call it "sundowning"; an unsettled or depressed behavior in Alzheimer's patients that usually occurs in late afternoon or evening.

Despite medication to relieve the symptoms, Billie suffers intense sadness. She stops crying, but her grief lingers. We sit in silence on the screened front porch of the home she shares with Frank. It's a balmy Florida spring day. Mockingbirds call and squirrels chatter in the eight oak trees. We watch Monarch and Swallowtail butterflies dance from flower to flower in the garden.

Billie begins to shake. "Frank is dead," she wails.

"No, he's sleeping." I reach for her hand.

Her voice quivers, "No, he's dead." Her eyes are wide with fear.

"Come with me, Billie." I lead her through French doors into the living room. Inside, Frank snores in his big blue chair. An unread book rises and falls on his stomach.

He looks so peaceful, I hesitate.

Billie whimpers beside me.

"Hey Frank." I wiggle his shoulder. "Wake up and show Billie you're alive."

"Aaah...oh...um, hello."

"Frank, are you okay?" Billie whispers.

"I'm fine, Billie."

Her face relaxes. "Thank goodness."

Frank smiles. He closes his eyes.

"Shhh." Billie puts her finger to her lips.

We return to the porch. Our neighbor Bill drives past in his blue van. He honks and waves. Billie smiles and waves back. She stares at the empty street.

"I miss my parents so much." She lowers her head into her hands. More tears spill from her eyes. She sniffles. "My dad was a lawyer. He worked to take care of us. My mom. . . she did the best she could. She tried so hard."

Billie's voice falters. I move closer.

"Your parents still love you," I say. "You'll be okay."

Billie sighs. She nods agreement. She wipes her nose on her shirt sleeve.

"Would you like to go for a walk?"

She says "yes" the third time I ask.

We stroll the neighborhood. We pick lantana, pet dogs, talk to squirrels and admire the purple flowers on the jacaranda trees.

We do this the same way, every day.

CHAPTER EIGHT

Adult Day Care

"She's perfect. She'll do great here."
— Pam

*B*illie sits on the bed and rocks back and forth. "Frank? Are you asleep?" She pulls his toes.

"Whaa?"

Billie's nocturnal escapades include rousing Frank at one, three and five in the morning. Days with no nights mean it's time to find an adult day care center.

Eleven months after I join Frank in caring for Billie, it's clear he needs more respite than the six hours I provide each day. Billie needs a full day of activity, without naps, to help everyone sleep at night.

The yellow pages, Neighborly Senior Services and the

local chapter of the Alzheimer's Association provide lists of nearby facilities that offer day care for dementia patients.

The first facility I visit is in downtown St. Petersburg. Traffic, potholes and puddles turn its parking lot into an obstacle course. Upstairs, in a medical arts building next to a hospital, signs lead me to a locked door. When I press the doorbell a thin woman with shoulder length black hair and thick glasses responds. She opens the security door and pokes her head into the hallway.

"Hello."

"Hi. I'm looking for adult day care. Can I get a tour?"

"Come on in. I'm Linda. Our director is in a meeting, but I can show you around."

A short hall leads to a large room with a gray linoleum floor and fluorescent lighting. A bank of windows are on the far wall. Two unmarked office doors are on my left. Half of the room is filled with a game of volleyball.

Twenty clients sit on chairs and wheelchairs on either side of a short net. They toss a pink balloon back and forth in slow motion. Aides guarantee the balloon stays in play.

"Do the clients go outside?" I ask.

"Sure," Linda says, "they can go downstairs for a smoke. We escort them to the parking lot and back."

"Oh."

"Well, sometimes we go to the park for a picnic," Linda says, "But mostly we stay busy here with crafts, games and exercises."

"Where do they eat lunch?" I ask.

Linda points to six cafeteria tables pushed aside for the

volleyball game. "We use those tables."

After the short tour, Linda hands me a detailed brochure that lists daily cost and hours. "There's a van that picks up clients in the morning and brings them here, then it takes them home again at the end of the day," Linda says. "It costs a few dollars extra. Right now we have a waiting list for it."

I thank her and say goodbye.

The next facility has a front yard shaded by three mature oak trees. There is a circular cement path and a patio filled with chairs. A four-foot high cinder block wall surrounds the yard, separating it from a busy street.

Inside, the receptionist slams the phone on its base. "Can I help you?" The abrupt woman furrows her brow and glares at me over her bifocals.

"I'd like information on your adult day care."

"Over there." She points to a pamphlet display. "You can look in there if you want." She waves at the tiny window in a gray door across the narrow lobby.

I peer through the glass rectangle. It's an identical copy of the multi-purpose room at the last place.

Next, I visit a day care center on a campus that includes a nursing home and Assisted Living Facility (ALF). It is called "DayBreak Adult Daycare Services."

Tracie, a thirty-something blonde nurse with blue eyes greets me with a smile. She hands me a green piece of paper. "This is our activities calendar."

Puppy visits, ice cream socials, crafts and balloon volleyball are noted on various days. A local beauty school provides manicures on the fifteenth.

"We alternate physical and mental activities. Patients watch a video during quiet time, or listen to music for stretch exercises," Tracie explains. We walk to the center of the dining area. "We also play word games and reminisce, to use our brains."

Eight round and rectangular tables, each with cushioned captain's chairs, fill the dining room.

"We use this room," Tracie says, "for meals, crafts and games."

Someone has printed on a large dry erase board: "Today is Monday, September 12th. Lunch is Polish sausage, mashed potatoes, green beans and bread."

Tracie says, "We have a continental breakfast every morning and snacks, too." She turns to face the hallway. "Let's look at the rest of the center."

DayBreak resembles a home, not a hospital. Except for the dining room floor, the center is carpeted. Teal wall-to-wall carpeting has a beige stripe that resembles a walking path. The path winds through the center. It guides pacers in a circle past the dining area, through a hall to the living room, then travels down a second hallway to return to the dining room.

In the living room, a gaunt woman with hunched shoulders shuffles to me. Her open mouth is in the shape of an "O."

"Ooohhh." She grabs my arm. "Ooohhh." Her unfocused blue eyes stare through me.

"Hello, how are you?" I ask.

"This is Jeannine." Tracie pats Jeannine's short gray hair

into place. "She's sweet and gentle, and never causes trouble, do you Jeannine?"

"Ooohhhh." Jeannine slides her feet towards the hall.

Tracie points to French doors in the corner. "Those doors lead to a patio and small fenced yard. When the weather is nice we open them. Then, everyone can wander in and out."

Six recliners, two couches and an entertainment center populate the living room. Paintings brighten the walls. Wood laminate shelves hold blankets, books and silk plants. Tracie shows me a second bathroom, then guides me down the hall to the dining area. A door from the dining room leads into the front office.

Dozens of white binders, each with a patient name on the spine, occupy two shelves above a built-in desk. "These contain daily records and vital information for each patient," Tracie says.

The office has a window that faces the parking lot, and a reception window that opens onto the lobby. We watch as a short brunette in a nurse's uniform arrives. Tracy waves to her. "Hey, Pam. This is Karen, she's looking for day care for her mother-in-law." Tracie continues, "This is Pam, our center director."

"Let's go to my office to discuss costs and services," Pam says. She leads me to her office. Tracie, an aide and the clients gather for "sittercise" nearby in the living room. Quiet orchestral music plays as the session begins.

"Okay everyone, stretch your arms to the sky, up we go. One, two, three."

Pam closes her office door. She points to a chair and I sit across from her.

"We employ two nurses, two certified nurse's aides and a social worker. Our maximum number of patients is twenty-four. We're here from seven until five-thirty, Monday through Friday." Pam recites prices to me. The fees remind me of kiddie day care costs. We'll pay weekly, based on the number of days Billie attends. The rates are reasonable—only a few dollars more than the other facilities.

Pam doesn't smile. "We also have a bathing service, available on request. It's eight dollars per shower."

"This is the first place that offered a shower service. That's great," I say.

"Yes. We have a walk-thru shower. A few of our clients use the service."

Pam hands me a five-page admissions application. "Just fill this out and return it."

"I want Billie and Frank to take a tour, too."

She forces a smile. "Sure."

"I'm curious to see how Billie reacts to this."

Two days later, Frank, Billie and I visit.

Pam greets us in the lobby. "Hello Billie! How are you?"

"How are you?" Billie asks.

"I'll assess Billie as we walk around the center," Pam explains as we step into the dining room.

Frank pauses to read the menu on the dry erase board. "Hmmm. I like your lunch menu," he says.

Pam laughs. "You can always join Billie for lunch."

A small, white-haired man with a pleasant, wrinkled face stands in front of us as we begin our tour.

"This is Bill," Pam says.

Bill fingers the buttons on his blue cardigan.

Billie moves to him. "That's my name, too!"

A smile flickers across Bill's face. "Yep, that's right." He reaches into his pants pocket and pulls out a spoon. He hands it to Billie.

After our tour Pam declares, "She's perfect. She'll do great here."

"Let's start with Billie attending on Monday, Wednesday and Friday," I suggest.

"That's fine," Pam agrees.

"Billie's son Craig will call you, too," I add. "He is legal guardian for Billie. He lives in Michigan. I'm sure he'll want to ask you some questions."

"Tell him to call anytime," Pam says.

Billie says, "This place looks like fun."

Pam smiles. "Will you come back and see us?"

"Sure." Billie grins.

CHAPTER NINE

First Day in Day Care

"I don't know what to do. No one tells me what to do."
— Billie

I stuff shorts, a shirt and socks for Billie's first day at DayBreak into an Audubon Society backpack. Just like a preschooler, she needs to take extra clothes to day care. One more item and we can go. I search closets, bookshelves, the cedar chest and hamper for one of twenty new pairs of underwear. Nothing.

Billie strolls past me and out the front door. Frank soon follows to retrieve her. I continue to search. In a minute, I hear Frank's muffled voice outside.

At the front door I ask, "What did you say?"

"Billie is far down the street. I can't catch her."

I join Frank on the front sidewalk. Our neighbor Terry approaches with his Labrador Retriever, Misty.

"Billie is three blocks away," Terry says. He strokes his dog's head and leans in Billie's direction. "Misty and I can track her if you want."

Frank pauses. "That's tempting. Well, no, I'm sure we can find her."

"Let's get her on our way to DayBreak," I suggest.

I run inside to grab Billie's backpack and paperwork, then Frank and I climb into my van. He surveys the neighborhood as I drive. We turn left after three blocks. Two blocks more and we find Billie.

"Oh my, look." Frank points. Terry and his canine hold Billie captive on the far corner of the intersection. The man and dog block her attempts to cross the street.

We pull to the curb. I lean across Frank and yell, "Hey lady, want a ride?"

Terry reigns in Misty. Frank slides open the van door. Billie hurries inside. Frank closes the door. I hit the door locks.

"Thanks Terry," Frank calls.

"No problem."

Everyone waves as we drive away.

Billie says, "He kept telling me what to do."

Frank talks non-stop during our ten minute commute to DayBreak. This prevents questions from Billie. Frank and I chatter as we exit the van. Billie follows us across the parking lot.

She touches the yellow hibiscus at the entrance. "What's this place?" She stops under the turquoise awning.

"You'll see, come on in," I say.

Frank opens the exterior glass door. Inside, we enter a door labeled "DayBreak." A chorus of cheerful voices startle us. Billie, Frank and I jump in unison. Framed in the reception window are Pam, a nurse's aide named Anisha, and Tracie.

"Hello Billie!"

"Hey Billie, how are you?"

"Good morning, Billie."

Billie doesn't recognize anyone, but appreciates their positive mood. She grins. The secure door that separates the lobby from the center swings open.

Anisha offers a wide smile as she holds the door. She towers over us, "How about some coffee, Billie?"

"Sure." Billie scoots inside. The door clicks shut.

Frank and I stay in the lobby. We turn to Pam in the reception window.

"Billie is going to love it here," Pam says. "She's perfect for us. Don't worry."

Pam hands business cards to Frank and me. "You guys go have a nice day. We'll take care of Billie. Relax, she'll do fine."

I drive Frank to his house. We separate until four-thirty when we return to DayBreak.

We scurry across the parking lot. "How do you think she did?" I ask Frank.

He opens the entrance door. "I'll bet she did fine."

We exchange glances and giggle. No one is at the reception window. I punch in the security door password. We peek inside and see Billie walk across the dining room.

"She looks good," I whisper to Frank.

"Yeah."

Billie's arms swing as she walks towards a table where Tracie and five clients discuss a stack of photographs.

"Hey, Billie," I intercept her, "Did you have fun today?"

"I think so."

"Good," Frank says.

Tracie reports, "Billie was anxious at first, but fine after an hour. She had a good day."

Anisha joins us. She pats Billie's shoulder. "I had fun today Billie. I hope you did. Come back and see me."

"Yes, fun." Billie looks around the room. "I'll be back."

Outside, I notice drops of orange paint on Billie's black tennis shoes.

"Did you paint today?" I ask as we cross the parking lot.

"Oh no, no." Billie shakes her head.

Frank asks, "Did you have fun?"

"Oh sure." Billie climbs into the van.

"Did you make new friends?" Frank asks before he closes her door.

"No, but I saw a lot of people I hadn't seen in a long time."

CHAPTER TEN

Trouble on Day Three

"I'm so lucky to be the person I am."
— Billie

This stern message is on my answering machine when I return from delivering Billie to DayBreak: "Karen, this is Tracie at Daybreak. Call me immediately."

Billie has only been there for twenty minutes.

I phone Tracie. "What's the matter?"

"Billie hit a staff member. She scratched me hard enough to break skin."

"No."

"Yes. And this isn't the first time," Tracie says. "There were incidents on the other two days."

"What? I didn't know that."

"The other times we were able to redirect or distract her."
I'm speechless.

"Pam wants to talk to you."

"I'm so sorry, Tracie. Billie isn't usually like that."

"It's okay," Tracie sighs, "hold on for Pam."

A minute later a voice asks, "Karen?"

"Yes."

"It's Pam. Have Billie's doctor prescribe an anti-anxiety drug. This is common behavior in AD patients, especially in a new situation," she says. "Although my staff is capable of handling it the other patients aren't. Billie's aggressive behavior isn't acceptable."

"Oh, man."

"Tell the doctor her behavior is sundowning. But tell him that Billie does it in the morning. She has a hard time in the morning, but is okay in the afternoon. Karen, do this immediately, or Billie can't return."

"Should I come get her now?" I ask.

"No, she can stay the rest of today. She's calm now. We'll let her stay so you can arrange meds with her doctor."

"Okay. Thanks." I put down the phone. I drive to Billie's doctor's office. In the waiting room, I tell my story to the nurse/receptionist. A few minutes later, I repeat it to the doctor.

"Billie needs help adjusting to a new situation. But, I don't want her doped up, that would be cruel."

This doctor caught Billie's case in the hospital emergency room last December. He isn't an Alzheimer's specialist, but he works with us. He prescribes .25 mg of an anti-anxiety medicine.

"It will take the edge off," he says. "My nurse will call the pharmacy for you."

Frank and I return to DayBreak at four-thirty. The staff social worker, Lee, is at the reception window.

"I want to talk to you," she says looking at both of us. She holds up a bright yellow paper with "Do Not Resuscitate (DNR)" printed in blood red ink across the top.

"You need to have this paperwork on file with us." She pushes the paper across the reception window counter top. "Alzheimer's is a terminal disease," she says, "Complete this form and return it to me. This isn't a Living Will. This is for the paramedics, so they don't resuscitate Billie if she has a heart attack or seizure."

I look at Lee's round face. The blue eyes behind her silver-framed glasses are serious.

"If we don't have this on file, to hand to the paramedics, they'll resuscitate Billie," she adds.

My throat closes. *What? Isn't that what we want?*

I look at Frank.

He nods to Lee. "Okay, that sounds important."

Frank and Lee continue to chat, but I can't hear them. I stuff the paper into the back pocket of my jeans just as Billie wanders into the office behind Lee.

She smiles when she recognizes Frank.

"I can't believe my eyes." Billie puts a hand on her cheek. "Look who's here."

"Come join us," I say.

I punch in the code, open the security door and lead Billie from the office into the lobby. She stands between me and

Frank and holds his arm. She smiles at Lee.

"It's important, you know," Lee says. "Alzheimer's is terminal. Get that notarized and return it as soon as you can."

In unison Frank and Billie answer, "Okay."

Tracie appears beside Lee. She explains Billie's physical outburst. "Debbie was filing papers in the office with her back to Billie. Billie tried to get her attention. When Debbie didn't respond, Billie slapped her."

Tracie pauses.

"I grabbed Billie's arms to stop her and she dug her nails into my forearm." Tracie turns her arm, palm up, to reveal four red and swollen half moon shaped wounds. The scratches match the curves of Billie's fingernails.

"Ouch." I wince.

"That looks sore," Billie says. She touches Tracie's arm.

On the way home, we pick up Billie's prescription. Frank plans to give Billie her first dose the next morning, Saturday, at home.

"If Billie has a reaction to the drug, we'll see it at home, not as a complication at DayBreak on Monday," he says.

Frank phones me at eight Saturday morning. "Billie is playing well with others," he jokes.

I visit an hour later. She is in a pleasant mood, but not groggy. Once again day care seems possible.

CHAPTER ELEVEN

The Struggle to Shampoo

"Don't you have someone else you can bother?"
— Billie

Inside the salon's front door she yanks her wrinkled hand from mine. "No. No!" Billie shrieks.

She swipes at the air as if she's drowning. Stylists and customers turn to stare. A hot flush of embarrassment climbs my neck.

"Okay, okay. It's okay, Billie."

I hug her tight and wait for her Alzheimer's-induced panic to pass. A quick nod to the curious, and we exit. Hand-in-hand we return to my van. I drive my seventy-three-year-old mother-in-law home.

Every day I say, "Let's wash your hair."

Billie crinkles her nose and rolls her eyes skyward. "I just washed it," or "That's stupid," she says.

After ten days without a shampoo, the comb slides out of Billie's hair on an oil slick. I try the beauty salon for professional help, but Billie's unpredictable moods sabotage four separate attempts.

On day eleven, I slip through the security door of DayBreak. In the dining room, Billie paces the shiny linoleum floor using baby steps.

She wears a green tee shirt and navy pants with her classic one sock on and one sock off, inside her black tennis shoes. The last fluffy spot on her head is gone. Her thick gray hair is a helmet.

She turns at the far wall and inches towards me like a slow-motion wind-up toy. A glimmer of recognition flashes in her eyes as I reach her.

"It been years! Where have you been?" Billie asks. She puts her arms around my waist. We smile at each other and hug.

"Are you ready to go, Billie?" I raise my eyebrows and nod at the exit door.

"You betcha." She positions her arms like a race walker. "Let's go."

Outside, she hugs me again. Her pleasant mood convinces me to hurry to the nearest hair stylist.

In five minutes, we enter the first-come, first-served hair salon. It's a large open space with fluorescent lighting. Stylists cut hair and chat with customers in the gray barber chairs along the mid-section of the room. Photos of multigenerational models with beautiful tresses decorate the walls. Hair product displays promise manageability. The smell of coconut shampoo drifts through the air with jazz music and salon sounds.

I look sideways at Billie. She taps her right foot and smiles at the room.

A tall, dark-haired man with a cheerful face approaches us.

"Hi. I'm Rick. Can I help you?"

"How long to wait for a shampoo and cut?" I ask.

Rick looks at Billie. "We can take her now."

"Wonderful." A heavy sigh escapes my mouth. "Would I be pushing it to have my hair cut, too?"

"No problem." Rick points his thumb at his chest. "I can cut your hair."

Lily, a slender stylist with a black ponytail, leads Billie to the sinks in the far right corner of the salon. Billie waves her arms and jabbers as Lily guides her into a shampoo chair.

Rick's fingers hover over the computer keyboard on the reception desk.

"Phone number?" He types the seven digits I give him. His eyes move from the computer screen to me. "Your zip code?"

"I should warn her." I frown. "Billie has Alzheimer's. She doesn't always make sense."

"Lily will work with her, don't worry." Rick smiles.

I recite my zip code.

We walk to the bank of sinks. Rick whispers in Lily's ear. She pumps shampoo from the dispenser and massages Billie's hair into a white lather. "Okay," she says.

Billie and I sit next to each other during our haircuts. Occasionally, she discovers me and says, "Well, look who's here." I reach over and hold her hand until she forgets.

Rick pulls a comb from an antiseptic-filled glass jar next to his award for styling excellence. He loops scissors onto his thumb and finger. He whispers as he trims my auburn mane.

"I was cutting a lady's hair. She had dementia, or something. We were talking and laughing. When I moved around to cut the back of her hair, she saw me in the mirror and she re-introduced herself to me."

Rick's blue eyes meet mine in the mirror. "She thought I was someone new."

Fifteen minutes later, Lily lays her comb and scissors on the counter. She swivels Billie's chair so she can see her reflection. Billie grins at her clean, stylish self.

"You look great." Lily says.

Billie looks again. "Oh? Yes, I do."

At the register, Lily calculates the cost of our visit.

Billie asks, "Is there a bathroom?"

"Go to the back of the salon," Lily says. "On your right, just past the archway, is the ladies room."

Billie saunters away. She greets stylists and customers as she passes them.

"It's the door on the right," Lily calls. She turns to me with a question mark expression.

"I'll let her try by herself first." I pull money from my wallet and hand it to Lily. I glance towards the bathroom and see Billie tug on the emergency exit.

"Uh-oh." I reach her as she swings her hip at the door. "No, no, Billie. Stop!"

"What?" She stops in mid-swing.

"Use this door. This is the bathroom."

Amid brooms, dustpans and stacked boxes of styling products, I wait for Billie to emerge. The handle clicks. I watch it twist and turn several times before the door opens.

"Oh, it's you," Billie says.

We wash her hands, then leave the salon. Halfway to the van, Billie grabs my arm. "What are we doing?" she asks.

"We just had our hair cut. Now we're going home."

"Okay, let's go." She puts her hand in mine.

In the car driving home I say, "Your haircut looks pretty, Billie."

"Oh?"

"Look here." I pull down her visor and flip open the mirror. I point to her reflection. "You'll see."

Billie's hands caress her hair. "Oh. Pretty." She turns to me. "I had no idea."

CHAPTER TWELVE

Support Group

"It's like the person you love isn't there. You find you're caring for a stranger with little or no help."
— Dan

There are eight people at the "Coping with the Holidays" meeting. It's a support group for caregivers of Alzheimer's patients who attend DayBreak. Two husbands, two daughters, a wife, Frank and I sit around an oval dining table. Lee, DayBreak's social worker, is our moderator.

"You have to realize what you're doing is hard, and you should talk about it," she says.

We're in a private dining room in the ALF next to DayBreak. It's decorated in rich burgundy and gold striped wallpaper and mahogany wainscoting. The room provides a civilized setting for our discussion of absurd behavior.

The first to speak is a man on Lee's right.

"Hello, I'm Dan. Some of you may know my wife Martha. She's the tall lady who counts all the time."

I shift in my seat to see Dan through the silk centerpiece of daylilies, ferns and yellow roses.

"Tell us about Martha and how you cope with the disease," Lee suggests.

A serene man with salt and pepper hair, Dan says, "Martha has had Alzheimer's for six years. We've been at DayBreak for nine months now. It's a great help to me."

Dan removes his navy blazer and hangs it over the back of his chair. "Martha loves to count," he explains. "I use her fixation to get her to eat, bathe and walk. We count everything." He shrugs.

At dinner I hold out the spoon and count one, two, three, then Martha takes a bite. When I give her a sponge bath, we count." Dan pretends to dab his arm with a sponge. "I count one, two, three, up one arm and down the other as I wash her. It works for us."

The next husband is calm, too. "I'm Steve. I guess we do what we have to do. I know Jean would take care of me, if the situation was reversed."

Steve has a thin crown of gray hair and thick glasses. His tan cardigan relaxes a white business shirt and navy dress pants. Steve says, "Jean got sick right after I retired. We had lots of plans to travel and visit our kids. They live in Ohio and Indiana. We won't do that now." He straightens. "It's too hard."

"Jean's been at DayBreak for two years," he says. "It means I can keep her at home. Since our kids live far away, I'm the only one to take care of her."

Lee smiles. "Millie, you're next."

Millie begins, "I am deeply hurt by our friends that don't call, family that doesn't visit or help, and comments people in my neighborhood make."

She draws a deep breath, then forces it past her lips. "We used to have a great social life. We went out to dinner and played bridge every Saturday. Now, none of our neighbors come over." Millie spits her words. "It's like they think they can catch it."

Around the table, every head nods.

"I feel like I'm in this all alone," she says. "And I'm mad at my husband, Ralph."

Millie is a handsome woman, with stylish gray hair and a fresh manicure. She wears a coordinated pants and sweater outfit. "This was not part of my plan," she says. "Listen to this. Can you believe yesterday Ralph had beer for breakfast? With leftover shrimp." She frowns. "I just can't believe some of the things he does. He drives me nuts. No matter how many times I tell him, he keeps doing it."

Lee interrupts, "I believe every word Millie says. Too many people do the caregiving alone." Lee points to the two men. "Dan has a daughter that visits when she can, and Steve has two sons, but they live far away."

Dan says, "It's sad. It's like the person you love isn't really there. You find you're caring for a stranger with little or no help."

The room is quiet. We all turn to the woman at the end of the table. Anna is fifty-five and single. She speaks as if each word is her last.

"I cared for my mother in my home for seven years." Tears escape from behind her frameless glasses. "Until two months ago, I worked at the veterans hospital in the psychiatric unit." Anna removes her eyeglasses. Dark circles surround her brown eyes.

"I retired three weeks before my mother died." She catches a tear with her index finger. "I cared for her for so many years, now that she's dead I have to learn how to live." She tucks straight gray hair behind her ears. "My life was literally on hold for her."

Frank pats Anna's slumped shoulder. She adds, "I've started to ride my bike and take long walks. I'll probably go back to work, but I'm not going to rush it. I'm going to take my time." Anna sniffles. "That's all."

"I think Anna is right about taking her time," Lee says. "It's important to grieve. It's time to pamper yourself. Coming here today is a good first step. Frank, your turn."

Everyone looks at Frank. He has a new haircut and trimmed beard. He looks rested.

"I'm Frank," he waves his hand at me, "and this is Karen. We're with Billie."

Millie interrupts, "How long has Billie been sick?" Frank and I look at each other.

"It was 1987 when I first noticed something was wrong," I answer.

Millie persists, "but how long have you had to take care of her?"

I answer, "She has needed supervision for the last four years."

Frank continues, "Billie and I go to lectures, the symphony, dinner, the movies. I'm not sure how much information gets into her brain, but it's something to do." He glances around the table. "Karen comes every day to feed us, and she takes us on lots of field trips. Sunken Gardens, museums, the grocery store."

I nod. "Frank and I are lucky because we can talk to each other about Billie. We both understand. It's hard to convey the absurdities to friends and relatives who aren't here. They don't realize that every part of every day includes Alzheimer's."

I look across the table at Millie. "I think fear keeps friends and family away. Some people don't know what to do, so they don't do anything. Not everyone can help."

Millie shakes her head. "No one helps."

"You can't take it personally."

Millie squeezes her lips together.

"Billie had horrible crying fits every afternoon. She would sob because her parents are dead, or she couldn't find her sisters or brother. Often, she thought Frank was dead when he was napping. I couldn't console her."

Millie nods.

I sigh. "Now that she's at DayBreak, she doesn't cry as much. The staff says she does well here. She's busy with the other people. She doesn't have time to be sad. I think Billie was bored with our routine." I smile at Frank. "It's a relief to have her in a place where everyone understands. That isn't true in public. Right, Frank?"

He laughs. "Billie loves to swat strangers on the butt in public."

Ginny speaks next. Petite and trim, she has reddish blonde hair and flawless makeup. She checks and re-checks the contents of her designer purse.

"I tried to cope with my mother while I taught aerobics classes and went to school at night. My brother refused to help. I thought I could do it all—take care of my Mom, my husband and two teenagers." She stares at her hands folded on the table in front of her. "Then I had a breakdown. I fell apart and couldn't do anything." Her voice catches. "Now, I'm trying to recover my life."

Ginny pauses for a breath. "I organized twenty-four hour care for my Mom. Today is her first day at DayBreak." She cries, "I feel like I lost my best friend and my mom. Like Millie, I think the isolation and the emotional roller coaster of this disease are horrible."

Ginny's tears flow in mascara streaked streams over her cheeks. She fumbles in her purse and finds a tissue and a mirror. Everyone at the table makes sympathetic noises while she repairs her makeup.

"I really do feel better talking about it," she says. "I didn't do that for way too long."

Lee says, "Well, in my eyes, you're heroes. All caregivers are, if you ask me." She smiles at each person. "The next support group meeting will be in one month. Don't forget the potluck Christmas party on the twenty-third."

Everyone rises. We saunter together to gather our loved ones from DayBreak. Ginny whispers a story to me and Frank as we walk.

"I couldn't believe it. Once, we were in a restaurant. Our waiter was really handsome. Mom was admiring him." Ginny grabs Frank's arm. "She told him, 'I wouldn't mind having your boots under my bed.' "

Ginny, Frank and I stand in a circle and laugh.

"I thought I would die," Ginny says. "She's eighty-five-years-old for goodness sake."

CHAPTER THIRTEEN

Kicked Out of Day Care

"Who else do you know who kisses plants goodbye and tells
them that she loves them?"
— Karen

"Hello. Hello?" Emily hands me the phone. "Here Mom, I
don't know who it is."

I put the phone to my ear. Someone is crying and there
are muffled noises. A desperate voice screams, "Why don't
you just leave her alone?"

I wait. Soon a voice asks, "Karen?"

"Yes?"

"It's Tracie at DayBreak. Billie is hitting and scratching
again. You have to come get her."

"Oh no. I'll be right there." I hang up the phone and grab

my car keys. "Billie is staying with us this afternoon until we meet Frank at four-thirty."

"What happened?" asks Emily. She's home for a study day during high school exams.

"Billie's causing trouble. I have to go get her."

It's calm when I enter DayBreak. Tracie meets me at the door. "What's going on?" I ask.

Tracie's shoulders rise and fall with a deep breath. "Martha has a cold. Anisha was helping Martha drink soup through a straw. Billie didn't like that, so she grabbed the straw."

Tracie leans against the wall. "Anisha asked Billie to move, so Martha could eat. Billie didn't like that, either. Then, Anisha asked Billie to sit down."

Tracie whips her arm backhand through the air. "Instead, Billie swung her arm and sent Martha's soup flying off the table."

I suck in my breath.

"Hot soup." Tracie squints. "Billie got very angry when we moved her to the front office to isolate her."

She says, "The excitement and confusion got worse. All the clients were riled up. Tony darted all around yelling. Everyone was crying and shouting."

"That's what I heard over the phone?" I ask.

Tracie lowers her voice to a whisper. "Yes. And while Billie was fighting us, she hit Jeanine in the mouth and reopened her cut lip. There was hot soup, blood and confusion. It was a mess."

Tracie and I walk down the hall to the darkened living

room. A movie plays on the TV. Anisha and Billie emerge holding hands. Billie is teary-eyed. She shuffles to me. We hug.

"You look wrung out, Billie." I put my hands on her shoulders and look in her eyes. "Would you like to go home with me?"

Her mouth silently forms the word "yes."

Billie and I hug three times before we reach the parking lot. We sit inside my van for a few minutes.

"Are you okay?" I ask.

"It was one thing, then something else." She raises her hands in the air.

"Yeah that happens. Don't worry, everything will be okay."

"I hope so," she whispers.

We drive in silence. I rub Billie's back. She pats my knee. Her sadness lingers until we pull into my driveway.

"I remember this one," she says.

"Yes, you've been here lots of times. We'll do a few things here, then meet Frank to go to the airport."

For the next three hours, Billie folds laundry, wanders our fenced backyard, attempts to walk home, folds more laundry, hides silverware, paces, tries to drink votive candles and asks questions.

"Can you take me home?" Billie asks repeatedly.

"Sure, after we get Daniel from school."

"I need to go home," Billie says. "Let's go. I have to go home. Can you take me home? I'm going home."

At three o'clock, Emily, Billie and I retrieve Daniel from middle school. We drive to Frank's house. Billie is restless.

Emily and Daniel stay at the house while Billie and I stroll the neighborhood. It's a sunny afternoon. We pick flowers, pet dogs and watch squirrels. We walk with little conversation for over an hour. At four-thirty we return to the house.

"Pam from DayBreak called," Emily says. "She said it would be best if Billie doesn't come back until after Christmas. If you have questions, call her."

"What?" I ask.

"She sounded nice about it. She gave me the message after I told her that you and Billie were on a walk."

"Billie's been kicked out of school?" I pace the dining room.

"No Mom, just suspended for a week."

"Oh no. Frank was finally going to have time with his sisters. Without day care, Billie may have trouble sleeping. Plus there will be houseguests. This is bad."

Frank arrives at four-forty-five. Billie and I are at the kitchen table watching Blue Jays in the schefflera tree outside. "Did you have a great day, Frank?" I ask.

"It was okay." He kicks off his shoes at the door.

"Well, I hope it was good. I have news for you."

Frank settles into a chair and smiles at me.

I blurt, "Billie was kicked out of school for a week."

"What happened?" he asks.

"Who got what?" Billie asks. She rises from the table and leaves the kitchen.

I describe the day's events to Frank. "I guess we'll go back to our old schedule. No more sleep for you. I can't believe she was kicked out of school."

"Do you think this will go on her permanent record?"
Frank laughs.

***

Two days later, I deliver Christmas goodies to the
DayBreak staff. Pam is at the reception window. "Can I meet
with you to get advice on Billie's behavior?" I ask.

"Yes, it's time," Pam says. "Come Friday at ten-thirty."

"Okay, I'll bring Frank, too."

Frank and I arrive fifteen minutes early on Friday. Pam is
bent over gift boxes and bright wrapping paper on a dining
room table. "I'll be right there," she calls, tossing brown hair
over her shoulders.

A lanky brunette hands scotch tape to Pam.

"Thanks, Norma."

Norma prances over to us. She stands in front of Frank.
"Isn't this exciting? All the presents?" Norma points to the
silver boxes.

Frank nods.

I smile, unsure if Norma is on staff or a patient. She
continues to stare at Frank. I decide she's a well-dressed
patient.

Pam finishes. Frank and I follow her into her office. She
shuts the door. We position our chairs in a three point circle
and face each other.

The clock on Pam's desk ticks fifteen seconds before she
speaks. "I learned this morning that our patient, John, is
leaving. He's been here five years. "So," Pam sighs, "this is a
day for goodbyes. John progressed to a stage where more

KICKED OUT OF DAY CARE

care is needed than his wife can give him at home." She squirms in her chair. "It's time for Billie to move to an assisted living facility, too. She's too violent for DayBreak."

Frank and I stare at each other, then at Pam.

"What?" I say.

"Martha was nearly poked in the eye, and Billie scratched Tracie's arms again."

"I didn't hear that part," I say.

Pam raises one eyebrow. "There's more," she says.

"What, more?" I ask.

"Billie kicks and hits the staff and other patients when she doesn't get her way."

"You're kidding." I look at Frank. His mouth is open.

Pam continues, "I've been in this field for a long time. I recognize the stages easily." She crosses her arms. "Families often don't realize how far along the patient is. I'm sorry if I've upset you. I didn't mean to be insensitive."

"I didn't expect this. We thought we were going to talk about increasing Billie's anxiety medicine." My voice catches. I swallow hard. "Isn't an assisted living facility a place where you're on your own? Someone just checks on you every once in a while?"

"Billie would require a secure facility, an ALF designed for Alzheimer's patients." Pam's fingers stroke the air to indicate quotations around the word secure.

"We weren't aware of constant hitting and kicking," I say. "I ask every day how Billie did. I didn't hear about a lot of this."

Pam looks at Frank. "I assumed it happened at home, too."

"No." Frank crosses his arms.

"Not at all," I add.

"Billie doesn't hit or kick us," Frank says.

"I can understand why it happens here," I say, "but at home, there are lines we don't cross. We know what upsets Billie and avoid it. We let her do whatever she wants, as long as it's safe."

Pam scolds, "That means Billie rules the roost. It isn't good to let the person with dementia call the shots."

She leans forward in her chair. "That isn't possible in a group setting. I need to be able to turn my back and know Billie won't hurt someone." Pam shuffles papers on her desk. "Billie is high maintenance. It's time to get help taking care of her."

Frank clears his throat. "On weekends, I give Billie's meds to her. One tablet first thing in the morning, around six, then a second dose of a half tablet around noon. Billie stays happy and calm. Can't we continue here if you followed a similar dosing schedule?"

"Isn't that what we discussed in November?" I ask. "We weren't told about these incidents, Pam. We thought things were going well."

Frank adds, "We could try making the second dose a full tablet."

Pam studies Frank's face.

"If Billie behaves, can she please come back on Tuesday?" I ask. "Long enough to contact her children and find an assisted living facility?"

The room is silent. The clock ticks fifteen more seconds.

We watch Pam's poker face.

"Okay. Billie can come back," she agrees. "We'll take it day-by-day. But, this is only until you find an ALF."

"Thanks, Pam." I shake her hand.

Frank shakes Pam's hand, too.

Pam opens her office door. Children's voices sing, "We wish you a Merry Christmas" to clients in the next room. We exchange false "Merry Christmas" greetings with Pam, then leave. We drive to my house.

"That wasn't what I expected, how about you, Frank?"

"Hmmm? No."

"Want an Irish coffee?"

"Sure."

Frank and I stare at the poinsettia tablecloth on my dining room table. Large mugs of coffee steam in front of us. We read our horoscopes aloud from the newspaper.

I have my own prediction. "This will drastically change your life," I say.

"Yes, radically." Frank gulps his drink.

"Everyone says, the family always has to be told when it's time. I guess that's true." I shake my head.

"I guess so," he agrees. Our eyes meet.

I whisper, "The worst thing Pam said was that Billie is a classic Alzheimer's patient in the final stages of the disease— a 6.8 on a scale of 7."

We sip our coffee in silence.

CHAPTER FOURTEEN

The Next Transition:
Assisted Living

"Everybody in this building is effing crazy."
— Resident of The Courtyard

*B*illie returns to DayBreak on January second. When I pick her up at four-thirty, everyone is in the dining room.

Bill, a slight man in a red sweater, sits alone with an issue of *Glamour* magazine on the table in front of him. He turns each page like a speed-reader. Snap. Snap. Snap.

Bill's blank blue eyes meet mine. His face is full of laugh lines, but no smile. Thin white hair covers his shiny head. His gaze returns to the magazine. Slender, wrinkled hands flip more pages.

Martha, the counting lady, pulls clothes from a green

laundry basket on the next table. Martha's light brown hair is styled and sprayed. She wears a beige pantsuit and sensible brown pumps.

"One." She plucks a white tee shirt from the basket. She folds the shirt and drops it on the table. "Two." A striped baby blanket is "three." Martha lifts a single black sock. "Four."

Billie stands at the far end of the dining room. Her shoulders curve forward and her head is down. Her arms hang limp at her sides. She pumps her knees, but her feet barely move.

Halfway to Billie, Pam sits between an emaciated man in a wheelchair and a petite woman wearing a turquoise cable-knit sweater. The man and woman are asleep. Pam looks ready to doze, too. She scans *People* magazine.

"Did Billie have a bad day?" I ask as I pass Pam.

"No, just like this," Pam nods in Billie's direction, "most of the day."

"Is Tracie here?" I ask.

Pam looks at her magazine and turns another page. "No, she's on vacation this week."

I move to Billie. "Hey Billie, how are you doing?"

She raises her head and stares at me. As I hug her, my nostrils flare. She stinks. Her adult diaper is not fresh.

I cast a disgusted look at Pam, then hurry Billie out the door.

"How long have you been like this?" I ask.

She doesn't answer.

At the car, I settle Billie in her seat on a pink beach towel.

I start the car and tune the radio to upbeat music. "We'll get home fast and clean you up," I say.

Billie stares out the window.

I pat her shoulder. "It'll be all right."

She nods. "Okay."

When we reach home, I yell "hello" to Frank's two sisters in the living room. Billie and I go straight to the bathroom and remove her dirty clothes. She sits on the toilet.

"What?" Billie frowns. She discovers remnants of toilet paper and a mess in her underwear.

"We'll clean you fast," I say.

"Oh my," she shudders.

Billie hugs my arm while I bathe her. "Thank you," she whispers.

"Any time, you know that."

We wash our hands together in the sink. I help her into fresh clothes. Frank arrives as I fasten the button on her pants.

A few minutes later, Frank, his sisters and Billie leave for dinner. Billie waves from the back seat of Frank's car as they drive away. Her innocent expression shows no memory of a bad day.

***

Billie's three grown children travel to St. Petersburg to help find an ALF. Her son, Craig, and daughter, Jenni, live in Michigan. They arrive together on Thursday morning.

76

Another daughter, Cheri, lives one hundred and twenty-five miles away in Ocala. Cheri will drive to town on Friday afternoon.

In the airport ten minutes after Jenni and Craig arrive, Jenni tells me, "People have been saying, 'I can't believe you're putting your mother in a place like that.'"

"Jenni, it's taken years to get to this point. Billie needs full-time care," I answer.

"I know, I know." She removes her glasses to wipe tears. "But it hurts to hear. It's hard enough already." Jenni, at forty-eight, is the youngest of Billie's children. She works part-time at a bookstore in Michigan.

"Billie deserves professional care," I say. "You have to be the adults now and take care of your mother." I give Jenni and Craig the latest issue of the local Senior Guide. It describes facilities and services. Craig compiles a list of places to visit over the next three days.

The next morning, Craig and Jenni drive Billie to DayBreak and talk with Pam. Later, Frank, Craig, Jenni and I meet at an Italian restaurant for lunch.

"What did Pam have to say?" I ask.

Craig's thin voice quivers, "Pam said Billie requires full-time professional care in a secure setting designed for Alzheimer's patients." He puts his elbows on the table. He clasps his hands and uses both index fingers to push his glasses up the bridge of his nose.

"She's right," Frank says. "A good thing is that Billie's socializing skills are intact. She enjoys everyone she meets."

"Plus," Jenni says, "Pam said that Billie doesn't remember

anything more than five seconds. So, she won't miss anyone."

Craig looks at his half-eaten pasta, then across the table at me and Jenni. "We have to do what's best for Mother."

After lunch we begin our ALF search at "The Courtyard." It's a gray stucco building that fills half a city block on one of St. Petersburg's busiest streets.

Charcoal paint accentuates the roof line and trim. Three gray canvas awnings hang over indentations that once were windows. The entrance is a glass wall with double doors.

Frank rings the buzzer/intercom on the left side of the front door.

A young man in his twenties opens the door. "Come on in," he says. His name tag reads "Ben, Certified Nurse's Aide."

The crowded lobby contains two worn brown plaid couches, a wooden oval table and five pressed-back chairs. The floor is gray linoleum. Six or seven animated patients, plus four people in various stages of sleep, populate the lobby.

A television blares from down the hall. A skinny bleached blonde stands next to it. She shouts into a phone, "I'm doing lots better. I'm gonna get outta here soon."

A red-faced man in his sixties scowls at us from the couch. He shakes his right fist and screams profanities. Streaks of dirt cover the sleeves of his tan windbreaker.

Jan, a brunette in a floral dress, arrives to give us a tour. She leads us away from the angry man and into the outdoor courtyard.

The belligerent resident looks me in the eye as I pass. "Everyone in this effing place is crazy." He throws his arms in the air for emphasis. "It's the truth."

Outside, there are four park benches, two oak trees and an empty flower bed in the cement courtyard.

Jan stands in front of us. "I'm sorry. He's drunk and really mad. Somehow, he locked himself in his room. He had to crawl out his bathroom window. We're waiting for the locksmith to arrive."

Jan waves her arm like a game show model. She indicates the stucco walls dotted with charcoal gray doors. Each door has a window next to it.

"This is a converted motel. As you see, all the rooms open onto this courtyard." She adds, "The rooms are large and have a private bath."

She leads us to an unoccupied room. A gold and green paramecium print quilt covers the bed. Matching curtains hang at the window. There is a simulated wood double-wide dresser, a closet nook and a small bathroom. Two paintings of Florida sunsets decorate the walls.

"Clients can bring things from home too, of course," Jan says.

"What about bathing and dressing?" Jenni asks.

"There are two nurse practitioners on staff and several CNAs. We help our clients bathe, if necessary."

"Not all the people here have Alzheimer's, do they?" I ask.

"No. Some of our clients are recovering alcoholics, others have mental problems and some have dementia."

As if on cue, a short bald man in a quilted pea green winter coat approaches. He claps his brown cloth gloves together and sings.

"Silent night, jingle all the way, oh what fun it is to slide."

He bows at the end of his song and leaves.

Next, a dark-haired man with a leather tool belt slung around his waist appears. He puts his arm around Jan's shoulders and smiles down at her. She says, "This is my husband, John. He's a great handyman. Right now he's fixing up my office." Jan squeezes him.

John nods. "Hello everyone."

"John and I are the new managers of this facility," explains Jan. "I work with the patients. John maintains the building and grounds. I'm excited to learn about Alzheimer's and everything else. I'm taking a class at the junior college."

Jan leads us inside to the dining area. "It's under renovation. We'll be done in another month," she says.

Drywall boards and cans of paint stand against one wall. Three round cafe tables with mismatched chairs are in the center of the room. A half-full coffee pot sits on a maroon counter next to miniature boxes of corn flakes.

Craig asks, "Do you accept Medicaid?"

"Oh yes," Jan says.

"What about walking?" I ask. "Billie loves to pace. Where could she move around?"

Jan leads us outside to the south side of the building. She points to a gray cement slab surrounded by cigarette butts and half-dead shrubs.

"This is where people smoke," she says. "If you look, you'll see a path that goes halfway around the building. Lots of our clients walk around back there."

A sandy trail made in the worn grass stretches to the back of the lot. The six-foot high privacy fence separates the yard from an alley and offices next door. Three splintered fence slats are on the ground near a gap in the fence. Jenni, Craig and I exchange distressed looks.

"That security code box on the gate means the residents can't get out," Jan points to the fence. "You need the code to open it."

Jan hands us her business card as we say goodbye.

In the parking lot, Frank says, "That's a fun place, and close to the house."

"I want a professional staff, experienced in Alzheimer's," I say.

Jenni says, "I didn't like it at all."

"Kinda creepy," Craig says. "Plus, we have at least ten more places to see."

"The rooms are isolated. Think about Billie waking up at night and walking into that courtyard." I look at Frank. "She'd be scared to death."

"Jan said they do bed checks every couple of hours," Jenni says.

"Well, there were lots of interesting characters," Frank says. "I liked it. And, they accept Medicaid."

"I think Billie should be in an Alzheimer's unit with trained staff. This place seems more confusing than calming." I point to five lanes of traffic. "Plus, what if she wanders into the street?"

Craig says, "I guess we'll look at more places tomorrow. Jen and I will go pick up Mom, now."

He climbs into the driver's seat of his rental car and rolls down the window. "Hey, Mom went to day care in her pj's

this morning. Jenni and I couldn't get her to put on clothes."
Frank chuckles.

"In her nightgown or pajamas?" I ask.

"Pajama pants," Craig says, "with her red Christmas sweatshirt and pink slippers."

CHAPTER FIFTEEN

Billie's New Home

"If we all contribute four hundred dollars a month,
Mom can go to Arbor Oaks."
— Craig

On Friday, Craig, Jenni, Cheri and Frank visit four assisted living facilities. I stay home.

On Saturday, I join the siblings for the third day of the ALF search, and Frank takes a break. We see two places in the morning, then stop for lunch.

Jenni wrinkles her nose. "Every place Craig, Frank, and I looked at yesterday smelled like urine." She pushes a cigarette into her mouth. "Except for Arbor Oaks. That's where we should put Mom." She flicks her lighter.

Craig turns to me and Cheri. "Its Evergreen Wing is specifically for Alzheimer's patients."

A huge jacaranda tree shades the patio of the Chattaway Restaurant in south St. Petersburg. Purple petals float in the breeze, then land on our plastic table and chairs. Pink antique bathtubs full of lantana and salvia separate the patio from the parking lot.

Jenni exhales a stream of smoke. "Can you believe Frank likes that first place, The Courtyard?" She shivers. "Yuck."

Craig says, "We'll take Karen and Cheri to see Arbor Oaks after lunch."

"It's beautiful and it doesn't smell," Jenni says.

"Well, I hope it's better than the first place we saw this morning." Cheri flicks a flower petal across the table. "That place was dark, smelly and depressing, and had no security, at all."

"And the other place," Craig moans, "too institutional with those linoleum floors and hospital beds."

"I could smell urine there, too." Jenni shakes her head. Purple petals fall from her gray hair. "Mom would be out those doors in two seconds."

Craig clears his throat. "A simple alarm isn't going to keep her anywhere. She needs a locked door."

"It just has to be Arbor Oaks," Jenni says as the waitress delivers three beers and an ice tea.

Cheri fluffs her short brown hair. She squints through her eyeglasses at her siblings. "You said Arbor Oaks is private pay. You said they don't take Medicaid."

An unseen droplet of beer splats on Craig's yellow polo shirt. He puts his elbows on the table and pushes his glasses to his brow. "We can go private pay. Mom can go to Arbor

Oaks if we all contribute four hundred dollars a month." He leans back in his chair.

Cheri says, "I want to see Arbor Oaks before we decide anything." She and Jenni order another beer.

Jenni shifts in her chair. "I'm not sure how much I can contribute, but Mom should be at Arbor Oaks." She takes a deep drag of her cigarette and blows smoke over our heads.

Craig coughs. "Right now, with Frank's contribution and Mom's social security and pension, there's enough money to last 'til October. Plus, with what we put in, Mom can definitely go to Arbor Oaks."

Jenni smiles. "You'll agree when you see it." She waves her cigarette like an orchestra conductor. "It's perfect."

Thirty minutes later, we settle into my car. Jenni asks, "Can't we get just one Risperdal pill, so we can bathe Mom?"

I shake my head. "A drug isn't going to fix that."

"Well, I wish there was something," she says. "Craig and I have been here four days, and I can't get Mom to bathe. She's had that red sweatshirt on for three days."

"It's not easy," Craig says.

"My friend who works at an adult day care in Ocala says lots of her patients are on Risperdal," Cheri says.

I turn the ignition key. "Just give your Mom a cat bath."

Jenni asks, "What's a cat bath?"

"A sponge bath. Bathe Billie with a soapy washcloth. You have to do it slowly. She'll say no, but do it anyway."

"I thought DayBreak had a shower service," Cheri says.

"They do, but Billie only had one shower there." I pull into traffic and turn north. "She wasn't agreeable enough for them to shower her regularly, so we went back to cat baths."

Arbor Oaks is at the end of a dead-end street. The two story building is reminiscent of old Florida architecture. It's set back on the property and landscaped with oak and ficus trees, hawthorne bushes and impatiens. A veranda sweeps across the front of the yellow building. The tall portico at the entrance has a green tin roof.

Inside, the lobby resembles a fine hotel. On the right is an elegant library with chairs and couches upholstered in deep green and burgundy prints. The furniture compliments simulated oriental rugs in the wall-to-wall carpeting. Full book cases stretch from floor to ceiling.

In the center of the lobby, a round marble top table holds a vase of silk lilies and ferns. To the left is a spacious dining room with a wall of French doors facing the front porch.

We wait in the lobby while the receptionist summons Susanne, the Marketing Director. A tall, slender woman with bright blue eyes and short dark hair strolls towards us. She smiles and extends her hand to Craig.

"Hey Susanne," he says. "We're back for another look."

"Good." She smiles at Jenni, Cheri and me. "I'm glad you came back."

Craig says, "We want Cheri and Karen to see the Evergreen Wing."

"Come on in." Susanne leads us to a door on the right wall at the back of the lobby.

"Arbor Oaks is two years old," she explains. "We offer the latest in ALF and Alzheimer's-specific facilities. This wing provides a secure, safe place for residents with dementia."

On the opposite side of the door, creamy beige walls contrast with teal carpet. The lighting is soft and home-like. A semi-circle of recliners and couches surround a living room area in front of us. French doors open to a back porch and circular walking path.

A woman with short blond hair and glasses greets us. "Hi, I'm Carol." She smiles. "I've met Craig and Jenni, and heard about you." She shakes my hand. "Would you like a tour?"

"Yes, please," I say.

"That's why we're here," Cheri adds.

"Carol is in charge of our Evergreen Wing. She will take good care of you," Susanne says. "Let me know if you have any other questions."

Carol shows us the kitchen/dining area. We stand in front of a kitchen with golden oak cabinets, microwave oven, coffeemaker, stove, sink and refrigerator. Above the sink, a simulated window provides an outdoor view.

"All meals come from the main kitchen, but we prepare snacks here twice a day." Carol points to the refrigerator. "Juice and crackers are always available. We bake bread and cookies with the residents, too. As you can see, this looks like a kitchen in a home. We try to make everyone feel comfortable since this is their home now."

In the open dining area there are six round dining tables, each with four high back chairs upholstered in seafoam green. Two small square tables with two facing chairs are next to the wall.

"I'll show you the bedrooms next," Carol says.

Cheri puts her hands on her hips and turns to Carol. "At

my center, I own and operate a day care center, we keep the kids busy and stimulated. Do you do that here? Do you have regular activities?"

Carol nods. "Yes. We have group exercises everyday, like stretching and walking activities. A couple of times a week we have arts and crafts. We have musical entertainment. Sometimes we go to a park."

"That's good. You have to keep everyone stimulated," Cheri says.

In the hallway a shadowbox is built into the wall next to each bedroom door. The box has three shelves and a plexiglass front.

"Since most AD patients remember fifty years ago, but not yesterday," Carol explains, "there are childhood pictures in many of the boxes."

Photos, baby shoes, figurines and postcards fill the boxes. One has a driver's license, another displays a bronze baby shoe.

Residents' names and room numbers are posted by each door. Wooden hand rails run the length of the halls. Bedroom doors are painted green while utility room doors are painted the wall color to camouflage them.

After a tour of the two residential wings, kitchen, dining room, living room, patio and backyard, we thank Carol and leave.

Later in my kitchen before dinner, Craig whispers, "Frank said on the way over here that he thinks we can keep Billie at home."

I point a spatula at Craig. "What?"

"He thinks they're okay at home."

"You guys have to be the grownups, Craig. You have to do what's best for your mom. It's time."

Frank doesn't mention his idea during dinner. He writes an e-mail to me later. "I'm in no hurry to pop her in a home. I think we can make do here quite nicely."

I reply, "If Billie had cancer you wouldn't deny her the proper medical attention."

Craig phones me the next morning. "When Lee, the Daybreak social worker, called to schedule our family meeting, Frank suggested to her that Billie stay at home."

"What did Lee say to that?" I ask.

"She said, 'Are you kidding? No way.'" Craig laughs nervously. "Thank God."

Two days later, Billie has a required admissions assessment by a geriatric specialist. Frank confides, "The doctor said the best thing for an Alzheimer's patient is to stay at home." He puts his hands on his head. "After everyone convinces me Arbor Oaks is right, the doctor says that."

"Frank, home care is what you've been doing for the past ten years." I pat his back.

"I have?" he asks.

"Yes. You cared for Billie at home longer than many people could or would." I hug him. "Truly."

***

On Saturday morning, Frank and Craig deliver Billie and a suitcase full of clothes to Arbor Oaks. At nine-thirty Frank calls me with the details.

"She woke up cranky at five this morning," he says. "I served her oatmeal, an English muffin and coffee. After eating she went back to bed. Two hours later, she woke in a much better mood."

"How was the drop off?" I ask.

"First, Billie didn't want to get in the car. Then, at Arbor Oaks, she didn't want to get out of the car."

"Oh no," I say.

"As we walked to the front entrance, Craig admired the impatiens and ficus trees. He asked Billie if she thought they were pretty. She barked, 'No.'"

I chuckle.

"I thought we were in trouble," he says, "but Billie followed us inside. When she saw the lobby, she said, 'fancy schmancy.'"

The nurse at the Evergreen entrance said, 'Oh Billie, we've been waiting for you. You're going to live here.' She hugged Billie while Craig slid the suitcase inside. Billie giggled and followed the nurse."

"Wow. Then what?" I ask.

"Billie was behind the door, and Craig and I were alone in the lobby."

The Snapshot Visit

"No one would help her out of the chair."
— Cheri

"She shows up, complains about everything, tells me I'm doing it wrong, what I should do instead, and then BOOM! She's gone for six months." Susan frowns at her leather boat shoes. "Oh she calls, but only to tell me what a burden Mom's Alzheimer's is for her. My sister is absolutely no help."

"Snapshot visit," I say. "We get them, too."

Susan and I are in the front row at a conference hosted by the Tampa Bay Alzheimer's Association. We compare caregiver notes before the "End of Life Ethics" session begins.

Susan smooths the wrinkles on her chinos. "Why do you call it a snapshot visit?"

"It's a tiny picture out of the whole movie. A snapshot. Family and friends come to town, see a fragment of the reality, assume they know everything, then criticize." I sigh. "They don't take responsibility for any changes they suggest."

"I think my sister is in denial." Susan pulls a pen and notebook from her purse. "She doesn't understand taking care of Mom means constant surveillance. I don't have time to paint the kitchen cabinets, for God's sake." She rolls her eyes. "I barely get through each day making sure Mom eats, washes and doesn't get hurt. My sister wants me to do home improvements, too?"

"Everyone's in denial in our family," I say. "Billie's kids think the right drug will solve the problem. They insisted the doctor prescribe a drug they heard about from a friend."

"Did it help?" Susan asks.

"God, no." I shudder. "I thought it was going to kill her. Two days after Billie started the meds, she was slouched in a chair, half conscious and drooling. It took me five minutes to rouse her enough to say a few nonsensical words." I ransack my purse for a pen. "The worst part is her kids insisted on the drug, then left town. They never saw the damage. They didn't watch Billie struggle for two weeks to recover."

Susan says, "My sister thinks she's involved. But, I'm the one who spends every day with Mom." She fidgets in her chair. "That sounds like I don't want to take care of Mom. I do. I just wish my sister understood what it's really like. Her suggestions make me so angry."

"I know. You do your best, then someone visits and tells you everything that's wrong."

Susan and I are silent for a moment. We watch a staffer place a bottle of water on the podium.

I snap my fingers. "Here's a good example. Last week, Billie's daughter had a snapshot visit at the ALF."

"What happened?" Susan asks.

"Well, first of all, Billie walks non-stop. Our main goal is to get her to rest, so she doesn't exhaust herself."

"Yeah, my mom is a walker, too."

"Billie was in an electric recliner in the ALF's living room. The chair elevates so her feet can't touch the ground. The idea is to keep her there to encourage her to take a nap."

Susan nods. "Makes sense."

"When her daughter arrived, two residents were trying to help Billie climb out of the recliner. The on-duty aides kept watch from the dining room about twenty feet away."

Billie's daughter got mad at the aides. She rushed to Billie and punched the "down" button on the chair. When Billie's toes touched the ground, they went outside to the walking path."

"No nap for Billie," Susan says.

"Right. Then the daughter complains to me. 'No one would help her out of the chair. Those aides should rush to Billie. I'm going to call the director on Monday and report them.'"

Susan sighs. "My sister's like that, too."

"She just doesn't understand," I say. "She isn't here enough to know Billie was in the recliner to rest. No one helped her out of the chair because they wanted her to stay in it."

Susan says, "I know people mean well, but it's annoying. Visitors get angry or sad, then blame everyone except the disease."

"You're right about that," someone cackles. The voice belongs to a silver-haired woman in the row behind us. She puts her bony hand on my shoulder and squeezes. "Hi. I'm Sadie. My husband Bill has Alzheimer's."

"Hi Sadie," I say.

Susan says, "Hi."

Sadie continues, "Our two sons visit once, maybe twice a year. They live in Chicago. When we talk on the phone, they say, 'Mother, stop cooking with aluminum pans.' or 'Mother, give Dad some ginkgo biloba,' as if that helps me." Sadie fingers the frizzy bun at the nape of her neck. "They talk to their Dad on the phone and think he's fine." Her red eyes reveal her exhaustion. "They think I'm overreacting. Ha!"

"I've been told that, too," Susan says.

"I think it has to do with soothing themselves," Sadie advises. "They want to make sense of a nonsensical disease. They want to control an uncontrollable situation."

"They want their mother, friend, mentor or companion back," I say.

Susan bites her lip. "I want my mother back."

"Visitors usually don't help," Sadie says. "They don't spend all the long days with the patient. They aren't living with Alzheimer's."

I turn sideways for a better view of Sadie. "Most people don't want to know how bad the disease is. Not giving gory details is tempting. On one hand you avoid confrontations, but on the other hand, you feed their denial."

Susan says, "I worry my sister won't ever have a good visit with our mother. When she does visit, she's depressed by Mom's decline. She can't appreciate the little joyful moments."

"I know," I agree. "Last week, my father-in-law and I were giddy because Billie called him by name. It doesn't sound like much, but it is."

Sadie nods.

A stocky white-haired man with a gold cross on his lapel ambles to the podium at center stage. He taps the microphone and clears his throat. He smiles at the full auditorium. Sadie, Susan and I turn our attention to him.

"We're going to discuss the characteristics of ethical dilemmas and end-of-life issues," he says. "As most of you know, families and patients have lots of different dynamics. The first is denial, followed by anger. The same stages as grief."

CHAPTER SEVENTEEN

Emotional Whiplash

"It's like a car wreck. People slow down and stare.
They comment from a distance, then figure
someone else will take care of it."
— Karen

It's the end of September, 2001. Frank and I sit on his screened front porch before a trip to visit Billie at Arbor Oaks. After nine months in the ALF, the sadness and anxiety that tormented her is gone. She sleeps and eats on a regular schedule.

Billie weighed one hundred and eighty-three pounds the last time I coaxed her onto the bathroom scale. Now she weighs one hundred and twenty pounds, which looks good on her small frame. Her weight-loss is the result of non-stop walking and eating three meals plus snacks at Arbor Oaks, instead of six meals or more a day with Frank. Also, weight loss can be another symptom of Alzheimer's. Billie is happy, busy and safe in the secure environment of the Arbor Oaks dementia wing.

"Craig called yesterday," Frank says, "he said there isn't enough money for Billie to stay at Arbor Oaks."

"What? How can that be?" I ask.

"That's what I wondered, too," Frank replies. "I thought everyone was contributing, like they said they would."

"Did you say that to Craig?"

"Yes." He nods.

I lean forward. "And?"

"He said, 'I can't believe you're abandoning Mother.' Then he said he'd call back, and hung up."

"Did he call back?" I ask.

"Not yet." Frank shakes his head.

The next evening, Billie's daughter Jenni calls me. "Craig wants to move Mom to Michigan, since Frank won't pay for her care." She adds, "I can't believe Frank is acting like this."

"What do you mean?" I ask. "You, Craig and Cheri promised to contribute money so you could choose Arbor Oaks for Billie. What happened?"

"I know," she sighs. "Maybe Craig and Cheri can afford four hundred dollars a month, but I can't."

I bite my lip to prevent words I'll regret.

"Besides," Jenni says, "I'd understand if Frank was broke. I know he wants to have money to pass on to his own children. I mean, I know it's his family money. But, it's like if your

Dad wouldn't take care of your Mom."

"How can you say that?" I ask. "You chose Arbor Oaks. You know how expensive it is. You're the ones who wouldn't consider less expensive facilities."

"Do you think this is happening," Jenni whines, "because Frank has a girlfriend?

"It's happening because no one contributed money for Billie's care, except Frank."

Jenni doesn't answer.

I take a deep breath. "Listen, there's no reason not to use Billie's Medicaid benefits and choose a less expensive facility. Billie could live ten more years."

"Well..." Jenni's voice fades.

"At least with Billie in Michigan you could spend time with her." I pause. "This is your chance to be with your mom."

"Yeah," Jenni sighs. "I'm looking forward to that. The facility Craig picked is in Saline. That's a couple of hours from me, but I plan to visit several times each week."

***

The next day, I e-mail Billie's children in an effort to make the best of her departure.

"Last night Jenni called to tell me that you are moving Billie...I can't imagine a better time to move her close to you. Billie is maintaining her weight, eating regularly and no longer has the

anxious edge that made life hard for her. . . .
Please let me know when Billie is leaving. I will
need a thousand hugs to sustain me until I see
her again. Please, realize that your mom is a
gift. It's not about how hard it is on you, it's
about spending time with Billie and loving her
as best you can, for as long as you can."

Craig responds with this terse e-mail:

"She is being moved because Frank won't/can't
support her anymore, after 24 years of partner-
ship. It is worse than death."

***

Two days later at Arbor Oaks, I find Billie outside her
bedroom struggling to put on a sweater. I straighten her arm
and pull up the sleeve.
An aide approaches us. "I hear Billie's leaving."
"What did you hear?" I ask.
"That she's leaving soon. I'm going to miss her."
"Did her son call?" I ask.
"I don't know," she answers. "Talk to Carol, she'll be able
to tell you."
"Okay." Billie and I walk down the hall.
Carol, the head nurse and unit director, is in the dining
room dispensing juice and cookies. She raises an eyebrow.
"Hi, Karen. What's going on?"

Billie pats Carol's back. "Hello. How've you been?"

"Fine Billie. How are you?"

"Did Craig call?" I ask.

"No, Jenni called." Carol hands juice to a resident. "What's going on with Billie's kids?"

"Well, here's what I know: Last January, when Craig, Cheri and Jenni chose Arbor Oaks, they promised to help pay for it since it's private pay here. Frank asked what his contribution was, the kids told him, and he gave it in a lump sum."

"Okay," Carol says, "so what's the problem?" She hands Billie a glass of juice.

Billie empties the cup in one gulp. "Thank you." She moves next to me and we hold hands.

"When Craig announced all the money was gone, Frank's lawyer said Frank couldn't contribute again until the new year." I swing Billie's hand. "Craig got angry."

"I gotta go," Billie says. She drops my hand and saunters away.

I turn to Carol. "It turns out, Frank was the only one who gave money. Craig, Cheri and Jenni never told Frank that they weren't contributing. He didn't know Billie's money was running out. Craig is power of attorney and legal guardian for Billie. Frank and Billie weren't married. So, Craig has been in charge of Billie's healthcare money. He manages the stocks and gifts Frank has given to Billie over the past three years. Money specifically for her healthcare."

Carol points to herself, "Jenni told me that Frank refused to pay, so they had to move Billie." She frowns. "She insinuated it was because Frank has a girlfriend."

"God," I say. "How can she say that?"

"I didn't want to believe it. It didn't sound like Frank," Carol says. "So, now what?"

"I don't know. Wait and see, I guess." I put my hands on my hips. "But if I knew there only was enough money to last until October without additional funds, you know Billie's kids knew it, too. I don't understand why they said they would contribute if they never planned on it. And why wait until the last minute to mention it?"

***

On November first, Frank shows me this e-mail from Jenni:

> "craig and i are flying down nov. 9th. he is still angry and wants to stay at a hotel, but maybe we can still all get together and have a pitcher of beer or two for mom and all the good times we all have had together. not sure when cher is coming down if it will be fri. or sat morning. we will be leaving on saturday in the a.m. or early afternoon. we want to get mom settled in before nightfall."

I ask Frank, "Where's Saline, Michigan, anyway?"

"Not far from Craig and Jane's house in Ann Arbor."

"But Craig works in Kansas City all week. Do you mean

he's moving Billie away from him and his sisters? The only relative nearby will be Jane?" I throw my arms in the air. "Jane, the person who is already caring for her own sick parents, raising their two teenagers and working?"

"Looks like it." Frank shrugs. "I guess Craig goes home to Ann Arbor most weekends."

"Explain to me why that is better than moving Billie to a Medicaid facility here in St. Pete? Near us, her regular visitors? Explain that," I demand.

"I can't," Frank says.

***

Three days before Billie's scheduled move, I'm at Arbor Oaks for a regular visit. As I enter the Alzheimer's wing Carol grins at me.

"Craig called. He said Billie can't be admitted to the facility in Michigan on the weekend. He'll call back when he knows when she can be admitted."

"A postponement?" I say. "That's good news."

Three hours later, Billie faints at dinner. An ambulance rushes her to St. Petersburg General Hospital's Emergency Room. She's conscious when I reach her twenty-five minutes later. Tests reveal she has a urinary tract infection. No broken bones. She is admitted for antibiotics and observation.

Frank and I chaperone Billie for the next forty-eight hours. We don't want her to be scared or alone. Plus if she's unsupervised, Billie will remove her IV and catheter and escape from her bed.

The doctor discharges Billie by nightfall on Friday.
"Let's go home," I suggest.
"Okay. Let's go," she agrees.
Frank chimes in, "Yes ma'am, let's go."
After a short wheelchair ride to the exit, Frank and
I help Billie into my van. We enjoy nonsensical conversation
and each other's company as we drive. For a few minutes
everything is right in our world. Frank, Billie and I are
together. It feels like one of the hundreds of field trips we've
made. A tear slides down my cheek in the dark.
Fifteen minutes later, we deliver Billie to Arbor Oaks. She
is greeted with smiles and hugs.
"How about some dinner, Billie?" someone asks. "We
saved your plate when we heard you were coming."
Billie takes a seat in the dining room, surrounded by staff
and residents. Frank and I sit near her.
"I thought she was going to die," an aide whispers in my
ear. "She started choking, then went pale." The aide's eyes fill
with tears. "I just love Billie. She follows me around all night.
She's so sweet."
"We were lucky," I agree.
Due to the side trip to the hospital, and her infection,
Billie's trip to Saline is postponed until after Thanksgiving.
Her daughter Jenni visits in mid-November. She confers with
nurse Carol and Billie's physician, Dr. Nuygen, who
recommend Billie stay where she is. Jenni and Cheri try to
convince their brother not to move Billie.
On November 25th, Cheri writes the following e-mail to
Frank.

"I guess there has been discussion between Jenni and Craig about $$$ to help keep Mom at Arbor Oaks. I believe Craig says he can do $300 monthly, and I'm not sure about Jen, probably the same or $100 more. Greg and I can do at least $400-$500, Mary Ellen said she can contribute $100.00 monthly too, with Mom's ss. ck and if you can contribute what you said I think we can do it."

***

In early December, Frank again contributes substantially to Billie's healthcare fund. Craig responds with this e-mail:

"The consensus is to leave Billie at Arbor Oaks based on the facts from Nurse Carol and Dr. Nuygen that it would be too traumatic to move her at this stage. They state if we move her now, she might likely die within three months due to the trauma of just being in a different environment. Also both stated she would likely not live through 2002, based on the facts that she is quickly wasting away due to the advances of the disease. At any rate, the decision to keep her at Arbor Oaks is a big one, and involves many factors. Her children have agreed to disagree with Frank, and contribute monetarily to her care monthly...."

"I wonder," Frank muses, "what her children have agreed to disagree about."

"Am I the only one who sees a pattern here?" I ask, "Why does he think any of this is new information? Why is it so hard to do the math?"

Three and a half months later, in April 2002, Craig announces, "There isn't enough money for Billie to stay at Arbor Oaks." Again, he suggests she be moved to a facility near Ann Arbor, Michigan. It doesn't make sense to traumatize her with a long trip, unfamiliar faces and colder weather. To avoid this, Frank gives Craig enough money to pay for three more months at Arbor Oaks.

Before Billie's kids come to St. Petersburg for a family meeting at the end of April, Frank suggests they reconsider a nearby Medicaid-accepting facility. He and Mary Ellen, one of his and Billie's dearest friends, discuss the situation before he sends this e-mail.

"I am sure the place in Saline would be very nice and closer to her Saginaw friends, but we were terribly worried about the trauma that might be induced by the trip. Especially in these days of augmented security. Long lines, shoe searches, body searches, etc. I think Mary Ellen put it best: 'Us old folks don't travel well.' Don't you agree it is time to reconsider alternative sites closer to Arbor Oaks or Ocala? As you know, the best care is most effectively insured by frequent visitation. We'll get an updated list of facilities that fit Billie's needs from the Alzheimer's Association. Hope this weekend will result in some good investigation."

During their weekend visit, Craig, Cheri and Jenni leave the list of local Medicaid facilities untouched on the dining room table. Again, they promise Frank they'll contribute money.

After everyone is gone, Frank and I drive to Arbor Oaks to notify them that Billie isn't moving. At a stoplight, I turn to Frank. "If money is the issue, why don't they choose a Medicaid facility in St. Petersburg?" I ask. "Plus, what do we do three months from now when Billie's kids say they are out of money again?"

"I hadn't even considered that," he says.

***

Our recurring nightmare surfaces for the third time on July 21, 2002. Craig reveals there is only one thousand, five hundred dollars left in Billie's healthcare fund. As soon as I read his e-mail I punch seven numbers on my telephone.

"That's it, I can't watch this anymore," I yell at Frank. "Eighteen months is long enough for her kids to figure this out. As soon as they didn't contribute, it was obvious we needed a place that accepts Medicaid. Not a place far away from everyone in a colder climate, but a local, Medicaid-accepting facility. Do you want to help me find one?"

"Okay," he replies, "let's do it."

***

Frank and I use the list of local Medicaid-accepting facilities we gave to Billie's kids in April. In under five hours, we find the perfect place. It's The Lodge at Mainlands.

CHAPTER EIGHTEEN

The Odyssey

"I'm so glad we got Billie. Now we don't have to worry
about her going somewhere else."
— Tangela

The next day I arrange for an assessor from the State of
Florida's Department of Elder Affairs to meet Billie and
review her case. Billie meets the criteria set by the state to
qualify for Medicaid. However, the waiting period for
acceptance can be anywhere between three months to a year.
Mainlands costs seven hundred dollars less per month than
Arbor Oaks. That's a significant and immediate savings that
will help until Billie receives Medicaid benefits. Frank pays
for the first month, and we set a moving day. Frank, my
fourteen-year-old, Daniel and I move Billie into her new
home on Saturday morning.

***

Billie grabs the backseat and hand rail after I slide open the van door. She attempts to lift her right foot to step on the floorboard and heave herself inside.

Frank looks in my direction.

Daniel asks, "Mom, can she get in by herself?"

"Oh, no. I forgot to bring the step stool." I climb into the van and face Billie. I wrap my arms around her chest and lift. "I'm going to pull, Frank, you push."

Billie giggles in my ear.

"Okay." Frank applies both hands to Billie's behind.

He shields her head as I lift her into the van. She's dead weight. She doesn't bend her knees or try to walk or offer any help. She hangs in my arms. Billie's hot breath hits my right ear over and over as I inch backwards. When her legs are in, I turn and fold her body onto the seat. I collapse next to her.

Frank laughs. "That was interesting."

I buckle Billie's seat belt. Daniel sits next to her. We drive across town to The Lodge at Mainlands. To extract Billie from the van, we reverse our loading procedure.

"Watch her head," Frank advises. He guides her feet as I bend my knees to clear the roof and lower her.

"Are we close yet?" I ask in Billie's ear.

"A few more inches," Frank says. "There, her feet are on the ground."

"There," Billie says.

In the lobby, a brick fireplace fills a wall. Plaid, over-stuffed wingback chairs and ottomans circle the hearth. We aim for the French doors with a purple floral print over the glass. These doors lead to "Heritage Court," the Alzheimer's wing.

I punch the four-digit entry code posted above the keypad. A green light blinks. Frank pushes and the door opens. There are rooms on both sides of the wide hallway. The roar of a vacuum greets us.

When the noise stops a blonde woman pushing the machine exits room 123. "You must be Billie," she says. "It's good to see you. I'm Chiara. Welcome."

"Hi," Billie says.

Frank, Billie, Daniel and I enter room 123. Bright morning sun illuminates the bedroom/bath suite. It's smaller than Billie's room at Arbor Oaks, but has a similar private bathroom with sink, toilet and shower. Mainlands is older than Arbor Oaks, but it's clean and has a friendly staff.

Tia and Tangela work full-time at Mainlands and part-time at Arbor Oaks. As we enter the hallway, they rush towards us and surround Billie.

"Hey Billie!"

"Billie's here!"

I watch as Tangela embraces her. Billie's little gray head nestles on Tangela's shoulder and neck, buried in warm brown flesh and long dark braids. Billie grins from ear to ear.

Tia and Tangela each take one of Billie's hands.

"Who should we introduce Billie to?"

"Merva would be good."

"Yeah, Merva and Billie could be friends."

"O-o-h-h Jay is going to miss Billie at Arbor Oaks." Tia shakes her head.

"Yeah. But, Billie and Merva will be good together."

Frank, Daniel and I follow for a minute.

"Hey, this is our chance to unload the car," I say.

"Okay," Frank says, "Billie is in good hands."

We return to the van and grab two suitcases, a package of adult diapers, a plastic bag of meds, a bedspread and pillow.

Back inside, Billie strolls by us with three new friends. Frank joins her while Daniel and I unpack.

When Frank and Billie return it's obvious she needs a quick change of her adult diaper.

"If you guys want to wait down the hall, we'll find you after we're done here," I suggest.

When we exit her room, I point to Billie's name on the plaque by the door.

"Do you know what that says, Billie?" I ask.

She frowns at the letters. "Is it me?"

"That's right. It sure is you." I squeeze her hand.

We pause in the hub where the two halls and common rooms meet. Daniel sits under a photo collage of family members, residents and staff at a recent gathering. Billie and I study the pictures and words.

"Faulty vissab," she says.

"Yep, family picnic," I read.

We walk to the back hallway and find Frank in a maroon wing back chair, reading a book.

Daniel stops next to Frank. Billie and I continue towards four residents by the glass door to the patio.

Over my shoulder I say, "If you want, I'll meet you guys by the fireplace in the lobby after I drop off Billie."

Frank rises. He and Daniel stride away.

Billie and I reach the group. They are discussing the security keypad that opens the door. A stocky woman in blue polyester pants and a striped pullover asks a frail woman in a wheelchair, "Do you know the code? Do you?"

The wheelchair-bound woman pulls a plaid knit shawl tight around her shoulders. She points a bony finger at no one.

A woman with cascades of white wavy hair says, "Your wife says you can do it," to a man in a red baseball cap.

"I don't remember," he says, and thrusts both hands into his pants pockets. His shirt looks like his morning coffee missed his mouth.

The wheelchair lady turns to the white-haired woman, "You do it."

"I'll try." She bounces to the keypad.

The man turns to Billie. "Do you know how to do it?"

Billie nods. "Yes."

"She knows," he yells.

The white-haired woman's index finger freezes in mid-punch. "Do you know how to do it?" she asks Billie, "Go ahead then."

Billie shakes her head. "I don't know."

The woman repositions her finger. She punches the numbers on display above the keypad as she counts out loud, "8-7-3-1."

The man says, "Now push the handle."

She pushes. The door doesn't open.

Billie doesn't notice when I release her hand. She watches

her new neighbors discuss who will punch the numbers next.

As I leave I see Tangela. "Billie's socializing down the hall."

Tangela grins. "She'll be fine here. I'm so glad we got Billie. Now we don't have to worry about her going somewhere else."

"Me, too," I say. "I can't tell you how happy we are that you and Tia are here. It's a relief."

Tangela says, "Yeah. I work full-time here and three nights at Arbor Oaks. I'm working there tonight."

"Tell everyone we said hello. See you soon."

Two familiar shapes lurk by the French doors at the end of the hall. A slight, hunched woman drives a cushioned black walker in circles around them.

"You guys are still here?" I ask.

Frank and Daniel grin.

I retrieve a cheat sheet from my pocket. "The director said one of the residents knows how to work the keypads, so they change the exit codes to stay secure. They don't post the real codes on the inside."

As we leave, Frank says, "That went well don't you think?"

"Yes." I sigh. "But, this emotional stuff is harder than physical labor."

"I agree," Frank says.

***

At ten-forty-five the next morning, I return to Mainlands.

I walk to the nurses station. It's sandwiched between the dining room and the back hall with doorways into both areas. Tangela is at a desk.

"Hi, I'm looking for Billie."

"She just walked by with Mildred," Tangela points to the back hall, "that way."

My eyes follow her finger. Billie shuffles hand-in-hand with a woman of the same height.

"Hey Billie."

Mildred and Billie look at me. Mildred's gray hair hangs halfway to her shoulders. Plump, pink cheeks mimic her round maroon eyeglass frames.

Billie and Mildred walk past me.

A voice behind me asks, "Are you Billie's daughter-in-law? I'm Mary, the activities director."

"Yes," I answer. "I'm Karen." We shake hands.

Mary explains, "I want to make an appointment with you to discuss Billie's activities and interests. We have forms we fill out with each resident's history." She waves papers at me. "It's so I learn about Billie's background and what she enjoys. Then I can invite her to participate in things she likes to do."

"Do you want to meet now?" I ask.

"It takes about forty-five minutes." Mary tilts her head. "Is that okay?"

"Sure," I say. "Let's do it."

"Okay."

Mary and I settle in the dining room by an open window. Outside, several residents walk in the fenced yard on a mulch path that leads from the side screened porch to the backyard.

Mary and I turn our attention to Billie's interests.

"Gardening?"

"Yes."

"Bowling?"

"No."

"Ice cream?"

"Oh, yes."

"Bingo?"

"No."

We discuss siblings, children, hometowns, animals, bird-watching, movies and museums.

Mary explains, "Every Friday afternoon, the residents go for ice cream. Last week we visited two preschool class-rooms." Her dark eyes dance above her smile. "That was a lot of fun." She shuffles her papers. "Another thing we do once a month is, I grab a bunch of burgers and fries and take everyone in the bus to Freedom Lake Park next door. It's only three dollars for the food, and the residents love it."

"Billie would like that," I say.

"We sit in the shade and eat. We feed squirrels and watch the swans in the lake." Mary adds, "Sometimes, I load everyone into the bus and we drive the scenic route around St. Pete. We don't get out, just drive around and enjoy the view."

A female figure creeps along the far wall of the dining room fifteen feet away. She heads for the pantry shelves filled with snack foods and paper products.

As she reaches for a gallon jug of fruit juice concentrate I call, "Billie, Billie, Billie."

She freezes. Slowly, she releases the jug, turns towards us and smiles.

"Come sit with us," I suggest. I take her hand and lead her to our table.

A table-setting crew of residents arrive. They bustle around the room positioning placemats, silverware and cups on each table. Billie moves to another table. She sits with three women and waits for lunch.

When Mary and I complete the paperwork, I stop at Billie's table to say goodbye. Her experience at Arbor Oaks makes this an easy transition. She knows the routine. Billie returns my hug and kiss. "See you later," she says.

At home, I cry for half an hour.

"Why are you crying?" my husband Charlie asks, "I thought you said everything went smoothly."

"It did," I sniffle. "It really, really did."

***

On day three, I take my daughter Emily to see Mainlands. "This is the infamous code keypad," I tell her as I punch the numbers.

We push through the French doors and stop at room 123. The door is closed. I turn the knob. It's locked. I consider the old fashioned turnkey bell in the center of the door. "Maybe her roommate is asleep," I say. "Let's see if we can find Billie first."

A staff member approaches us. "Billie and I were just naming fish down the hall."

Billie, in pink slacks and matching striped shirt, is near the fish tank. She laughs when she sees us.

"Want to show Emily around this place?" I ask.

"Sure," Billie says.

As we walk, Emily and I listen to two ladies in front of us. They are hatching a plan "to get the car."

"Well, what should we do when we find it?" the first one asks. She wrings her hands.

Her cohort replies, "We'll have to do something 'cause he won't get it right."

They nod at each other. They whisper and walk on. We pass them fifteen minutes later, and the plan is at the same stage of development.

At the patio door Emily says, "This yard is cozier than Arbor Oaks. There's more shade."

Two porch swings, a picnic table with umbrella, a decorative water fountain made of urns, and a shaded cement patio full of green plastic chairs looks inviting.

Billie is alert today. Each time we think she'll forget us and wander away, she turns, smiles and waits until we are together again.

I ask an aide about the locked bedroom door. "Did that happen accidentally?"

"With some of the nicer rooms they lock the doors so residents don't move someone else's belongings. But, it happens anyway," she says.

Billie's roommate, Sarah, has a television and lots of possessions from home in their room. Billie has her clothes, a photo album and facility-issued furniture. The aide unlocks the door so we can show the room to Emily.

As we enter Billie says, "Oh, this is nice."

Emily agrees, "It's smaller than Arbor Oaks, but Billie's never in her room anyway."

We return to the dining area at four forty-five. We see some people claiming their places for the evening meal.

"Why don't you sit here for dinner, Billie?" I help her into a chair. "We'll see you soon." I kiss her cheek and pat her back.

A short, unnaturally black-haired lady with wrinkles like rivers blocks me when I turn to leave.

One hand on her hip, she points to her cheek. She says, "Aren't you forgetting something?"

I peck her cheek. She smiles and walks away.

Emily and I head home. "Lots of the residents seem in an earlier stage of Alzheimer's than Billie," Emily says.

"That should stimulate her, I think." I smile. "I can't help but think her giggly mood is from the fun of meeting new people and exploring a new place."

Emily nods. "She was happy, that's for sure."

CHAPTER NINETEEN

A Bedtime Story

"It just doesn't matter one little bit."
— Billie

Billie's profile reminds me of Neanderthal man. A lump protrudes from her normally flat forehead. She lies on her back under a quilted pink bedspread, unaware that she's hurt.

Billie tumbled in the unfamiliar garden of her new Alzheimer's assisted living facility. Two tiny scrapes on one hand and a nickel-sized brush burn on her knee prove her forehead stopped the fall.

Shadows creep into the bedroom as daylight fades outside. Across the room a television murmurs and glows from its perch on a low dresser.

My watch snags a loose thread on the bedspread as I rearrange it over Billie's frail seventy-five-year-old body. "Where's your bedspread, Billie? I saw it in a room down the hall yesterday."

She smiles at my jovial tone. "It just doesn't matter one little bit." She pats my forearm.

I smile, too. "You're right, it doesn't matter."

I move a green metal chair with a fake bamboo back next to her bed. She pulls herself onto her elbows to watch my face by the light of the television.

"Lie down. You need to rest."

She doesn't move.

"Put your head here." I pat the plump white pillow, then lift and straighten each elbow so she reclines. "Try to sleep." I stroke her short, thick, gray hair, then study her thin, wrinkled face and lost eyes.

Billie extends her arm. She puts her cold palm on my cheek. "Oh, poor Billie," she says.

"If I tuck you in, will you sleep?" I fold her arms across her chest and push the pink coverlet around her body.

She sighs.

I sit down, put my feet on her bed and lean back. Metal bamboo pinches my spine. I watch the flickering figures on TV. A public television membership drive returns to the featured program: Dr. Perricone's lecture on healthy aging and his new book, *The Perricone Prescription*. Twenty minutes into the doctor's presentation, Billie is asleep.

The television brightens when the doctor and a female announcer pose in front of animated volunteers on a phone bank.

The announcer says, "Our volunteers are anxious to take your calls." She grins at the camera. "Remember, with your membership you'll receive Dr. Perricone's first book, *The Wrinkle Cure*, plus the lecture video, plus his new book, *The Perricone Prescription*."

Dr. Perricone nods. "And, I promise my plan will improve your clear thinking and youthfulness in twenty-eight days."

Billie's eyelashes flutter in REMs. I wonder what she dreams. Does she think clearly in her dreams? Does she remember names and faces and places? Does she know who she is?

On the television, Dr. Perricone explains why multi-syllable supplements maintain youth. Before the final commercial break, he aims his steady gaze at the camera. "When we come back, I'll tell you how you can get a facelift using natural methods."

The camera pans to a wrinkle-free blonde woman in the studio audience. She raises her eyebrows and scribbles on a notepad.

Billie sleeps. I rise and tiptoe out of the room. I don't wait for the TV doctor to return.

It just doesn't matter one little bit.

CHAPTER TWENTY

Heart Strings

"I'm moving Mother to Kansas City in six days."
— Craig

An invisible heart string connects me to Billie. I imagine it as a pulsating neon filament that stretches from my heart to hers. Our connection, looped and knotted several times for safety, buzzes and glows with each happiness and hardship we share.

When Billie is sad or hurt the string twists into a ball and drops like a weight in my stomach. Sometimes it catches in my throat or tugs at my heart. Today, pulled taunt enough for a tightrope, it hurts.

"I'm moving Mother to Kansas City in six days," her son Craig writes in an e-mail, "to a Medicaid nursing home."

Billie doesn't feel distress like me. She paces the assisted living facility as usual. She pauses to pat shoulders and socialize with the twenty words left in her vocabulary. Lost inside her diminished body, she's unaware of her travel plans.

My moist eyes study Billie as she naps. I'm determined to remember every detail. Lying on her back she resembles a malnourished mountain range. Her pointed nose and sharp chin are peaks above the valley of her sunken chest. Hip bones protrude to join twin knees as mountains. Her toes, mangled by a life spent barefoot, complete the terrain with a foothill. There are no mountains in the flat plains of Kansas City, Missouri.

"Where are they taking her? What is the address and phone number?" I ask Frank.

Craig provides only the name. An internet search reveals the facility is on the National Nursing Home Watch List. There is a reprimand for two recent violations of "actual harm and immediate danger" to residents.

Craig exercises the rights of a legal guardian. He decides to relocate Billie two months after she moved into Mainlands. My heart strings can't stop him.

Billie rises to pace again. As she walks away, I admit our heart string won't reach from here in Florida to Kansas City. When Billie's threadbare memory forgets our bond, I'll reconnect with a string of tears.

ALZHEIMER'S STORIES

124

Epilogue

Despite the heartache, Alzheimer's Disease taught me many wonderful lessons.

Here are my favorites:

- If you can't find something, check the freezer.

- Live in the moment.

- Don't worry about appearance.

- More than half the people you talk to won't realize your patient isn't making sense.

- Where you are isn't always where you think you are.

- It's good to forget what made you mad, sad or upset.

- Old memories are the best.

- Any and all food can be eaten in the middle of the night or for breakfast.

- If you can't find both socks, just wear one.

- Names don't matter, but emotions do.

- If it doesn't work now, try again in five minutes.

- Ask for help. You may not get it, but then again, you might.

- No one likes to be told what to do.

- There is tremendous beauty in every day life.

- Smile a lot. It makes everyone feel better.

- Reality and reason can be suspended without consequence.

- If you feel safe and loved, you're okay. If you make someone else feel safe and loved, you're living your life.

ALZHEIMER'S STORIES

Appendix A

The Ten Warning Signs of Alzheimer's Disease

with Examples of Billie's Behaviors

The following checklist of ten common symptoms, developed by the Alzheimer's Disease and Related Disorders Association, can help you recognize signs of Alzheimer's Disease. If someone you know has more than one of these symptoms, the Association recommends a visit to a physician.

Website for the United States Alzheimer's Association:
http://www.alz.org

Website for Alzheimer's Disease International:
http://www.alz.co.uk

Ten Warning Signs of Alzheimer's Disease.
Copyright 2003. Alzheimer's Disease and Related Disorders Association, Inc. All Rights Reserved. (http://www.alz.org)

1. **Memory loss.**
2. **Difficulty performing familiar tasks.**
3. **Problems with language.**
4. **Disorientation of time and place.**
5. **Poor or decreased judgment.**
6. **Problems with abstract thinking.**
7. **Misplacing things.**
8. **Changing in mood or behavior.**
9. **Changes in personality.**
10. **Loss of Initiative.**

1. Recent memory loss that affects job skills.

It's normal to occasionally forget names, dates, places. Most people remember them later. A person with Alzheimer's Disease may forget often and never remember them later.

What Billie Did: In the early stages of Alzheimer's, she forgot where we were going, where to meet, or what planned activity was next.

Mid-way through the disease, Billie answered the telephone and told the caller to "hold on." Then, she wandered the house with the phone in her hand. Minutes later, she rediscovered the phone and disconnected. Sometimes it would take five attempts to reach Frank by phone if Billie was first to answer.

During late-stage Alzheimer's, Billie's memory span decreased to five-ten seconds. She forgot the person whose hand she held. She often was surprised to see the person she spoke to seconds earlier.

2. Difficulty performing familiar tasks.

Busy people can be distracted from time to time. They may leave the carrots on the stove and only remember to serve them at the end of the meal. People with Alzheimer's could prepare a meal and not only forget to serve it, but also forget they made it.

What Billie Did: Billie would mix edibles and non-edibles when preparing food. The scariest combination was a sandwich made with pumice soap and peanut butter.

Billie often forgot she had eaten. This resulted in non-stop meals and weight gain.

3. Problems with language.

Everyone has trouble finding the right word sometimes, but a person with Alzheimer's may forget simple words or substitute inappropriate words, making his or her sentence incomprehensible.

What Billie Did: Mixed up words. Early in the disease, Billie recognized that she used the wrong words. She commented, "Oh, don't listen to me, I'm crazy."

Often like-sounding words were confused. For example, "roof" became "Ruth." As in "roofs? Is he talking about my sister, Ruth?"

Eventually, Billie stopped correcting herself and was unaware of confused or inappropriate conversation.

4. Disorientation of time and place.

It's normal to forget the day of the week or your destination for a moment. But people with Alzheimer's Disease can become lost on their own street, not knowing where they are, how they got there, or how to get back home.

What Billie Did: Billie constantly asked, "Where are we? Where are we going?" A common request was "Can you take me home?"

Once in the car Billie asked, "Where are we?"

"St. Petersburg, Florida," I replied.

"It's easy," she said, "to see things once you know where you are."

5. Poor or decreased judgement.

People can become so immersed in an activity that they temporarily forget the child they're watching. People with

Alzheimer's could forget entirely the child under their care. Also, they may dress inappropriately for weather or situations.

What Billie Did: Billie would insist on wearing a sweatshirt and jacket on hot days, or a T-shirt and no jacket on cold days. Once she wore a nightshirt to dinner at our house.

Billie constantly moved furniture in the side yard. She used all her energy to cram lawn chairs and tables into a full utility shed for no reason.

6. Problems with abstract thinking.

Balancing a checkbook may be disconcerting when the task is more complicated than usual. Someone with Alzheimer's Disease could forget completely what the numbers are and what needs to be done with them.

What Billie Did: Billie would randomly dial numbers on the phone or answer it when it didn't ring. She would write nonsensical messages in odd places before we left the house. Once she wrote across a newspaper: "We are here and we'll be back" then she threw the newspaper in the wastebasket.

7. Misplacing things.

Anyone can temporarily misplace a wallet or keys. But, a person with Alzheimer's may put things in inappropriate places: such as an iron in the freezer or a wristwatch in the sugar bowl.

What Billie Did: One of our biggest challenges was putting away groceries. By the time we unloaded the car, Billie would have the ice cream on the back porch and cereal in the bedroom. I learned to keep her busy carrying one small item at a time from the car to the house while I put groceries away.

Frank kept a "Missing in Action" list posted on the fridge for items we hoped to find. We learned not to leave anything valuable unattended because not only was Billie good at hiding items, she was fast about taking them.

8. Changes in mood or behavior.

Everyone becomes sad or moody from time to time. Someone with Alzheimer's can exhibit rapid mood swings—from calm to tears to anger—for no apparent reason.

What Billie Did: Billie was sad every afternoon and evening. Often she would wake in the middle of the night and be frightened and disoriented. She experienced intense grief for her parents. It took concentrated efforts to distract Billie into a new thought or to cheer her.

9. Changes in personality.

People's personalities ordinarily change somewhat with age. But a person with Alzheimer's Disease can change drastically, becoming extremely confused, suspicious or fearful.

What Billie Did: Billie experienced confusion, anxiety and intense fear when she imagined "bad people" in the house. Kind, thoughtful neighbors helped many times. When Billie knocked on their doors late at night, full of fear, they escorted her home, checked the house, and woke Frank.

Billie grew angry and uncooperative during her time in day care. I believe that was because she was unhappy with the situation, but couldn't tell us.

10. Loss of initiative.

It's normal to tire of housework, business activities or social obligations, but most people regain their initiative. The person with Alzheimer's Disease may become very passive and require cues and prompting to become involved.

What Billie Did: Billie wandered aimlessly. She searched for a familiar activity. She told Frank, "I don't know what I'm supposed to do. No one tells me what to do." When she didn't find something to occupy her, Billie would sleep.

Often Billie took three or four naps a day, more if she felt sad. This was terrible because it disturbed her nighttime sleep patterns. She kept herself and Frank awake most of the night. They were both exhausted. Day care and assisted living improved this situation.

ALZHEIMER'S STORIES

ACKNOWLEDGMENTS

Thank you, Jeri Fayad, for your passionate belief in this book. You made me believe, too.

Love and thanks to my parents, family and friends for making me feel safe and loved.

Special thanks to Bobbi Lurie, a fellow caregiver who shared this surreal path with me in conversation and spirit. I cherish our synchronicity.

Endless gratitude to everyone in Flash Memoirs. Your feedback and encouragement made it possible to tell this story.

Thanks to Anne Favo for jump-starting the editing process, and to Dr. Bob Rich for continuing it.

Warm wishes to all caregivers who do what has to be done. You are beautiful.

Contact the author:
Alzheimers_Stories@yahoo.com

Sign up for our monthly Alzheimer's newsletter:
Alzheimers_Stories-subscribe@yahoogroups.com

Order additional copies of this publication
in electronic or print format:
www.booklocker.com